Postmodern and Poststructural Approaches to Nursing Research

Postmodern and Poststructural Approaches to Nursing Research

Julianne Cheek

Sage Publications, Inc.
International Educational and Professional Publisher
Thousand Oaks ▪ London ▪ New Delhi

For information:

 Sage Publications, Inc.
2455 Teller Road
Thousand Oaks, California 91320
E-mail: order@sagepub.com

Sage Publications Ltd.
6 Bonhill Street
London EC2A 4PU
United Kingdom

Sage Publications India Pvt. Ltd.
M-32 Market
Greater Kailash I
New Delhi 110 048 India

Printed in the United States of America

Library of Congress Cataloging-in-Publication Data

Cheek, Julianne.
  Postmodern and poststructural approaches to nursing research /
by Julianne Cheek.
    p. cm.
  Includes bibliographical references and index.
  ISBN 0-7619-0674-6 (cloth: acid-free paper)
  ISBN 0-7619-0675-4 (pbk.: acid-free paper)
    1. Nursing—Research. 2. Postmodernism. 3. Poststructuralism. I.
Title.
  RT81.5 .C486 1999
  610.73'07'2—dc21   99-6366

This book is printed on acid-free paper.

00 01 02 03 04 05 06 7 6 5 4 3 2 1

Acquisition Editor: Dan Ruth
Editorial Assistant: Anna Howland
Production Editor: Diana E. Axelsen
Editorial Assistant: Nevair Kabakian

Contents

Preface

We hear and read the terms *postmodern* and *poststructural* with increasing frequency in the nursing and health care arenas. Yet their increased usage has not necessarily meant that these terms are well understood, nor that their potential for contributing to research endeavors in the health field is recognized. This was one of the reasons I decided to embark on writing a book such as this. I wanted to show that postmodern and poststructural approaches to research do not have to be obscure, ambiguous or poorly understood. Rather, I believe that some of the criticism of these approaches in terms of their inaccessibility and unintelligibility stems from a lack of definition or even at times the poor scholarship with which they are used and discussed.

Secondly, I had experienced both rejection of papers I had prepared for journals, and difficulty in attracting funding for research using these approaches. This led me to question why this was so. What assumptions were being made about research and scholarship that seemed to preclude writing and researching within these frameworks? Was the rejection of a paper, for example, based on what it said, how it said it, what it didn't say and/or assumptions about what it should say? Much of the discussion to follow in this book shares with readers my exploration of such questions and where it has led me.

The book makes no claim to providing definitive answers about either these issues or postmodern and poststructural approaches. Rather, it provides a beginning point from which readers can embark on their own journey of exploration of the potential afforded nursing and health care by these approaches.

I have attempted to write the book in an accessible and user-friendly way. I hope that you, the reader, are able to engage with the material and that the further readings suggested assist you to develop your understandings of postmodern and poststructural research approaches. Use the book as a "critical friend" in your journey of exploration.

Acknowledgments

I would like to acknowledge, with thanks, the role that the following people have played in the production of this book:

- The Faculty of Nursing, University of South Australia, for supporting this project.
- Julie Henderson, who has provided research assistance throughout the entire creation of the book. She has been meticulous in assisting with referencing, gaining permissions, editing manuscripts, proofreading and obtaining seemingly unobtainable references!
- Melanie Tucker, who has provided backup research assistance. Her proofreading skills have also been greatly appreciated, particularly at the final stages of the project.
- Irene Doskatsch, who has provided, and continues to provide, outstanding assistance in the library.
- Sage (London), Blackwell Science Asia, Allen & Unwin, *The Advertiser* and The University of South Australia for granting permission to use material in various sections of the book.
- The three anonymous reviewers who provided important and useful feedback on the first draft of the manuscript.
- Finally, sincere thanks to my family for their forebearance in the light of tight deadlines and broken wrists!

Chapter 1

Setting The Parameters:
What This Book Is About And Why It Is Important

THIS BOOK AS A RESPONSE TO RESEARCH IN NURSING/HEALTH CARE AS AN EVOLVING PROCESS

Contemporary nursing literature has increasingly urged nurses to embrace research as a core feature of their professional role. Research refers to "original, creative intellectual activity leading to the generation of new knowledge" (Whitworth 1994, p. 26). Such calls have developed from a growing awareness of the way in which research findings can inform practice and assist nurses and other health care practitioners to grapple with the demands of an increasingly diverse and complex professional role in late twentieth century society.

Yet such an evolving interest in research has not been without problems. Not least among the issues to emerge is the question of what constitutes both "legitimate" research subject matter and appropriate ways of researching particular issues in the health arena. As Dzurec (1989) notes: "The human sciences, including nursing, have a long tradition of struggling with the problem of identifying an appropriate conceptual framework and methods for the conduct of research" (p. 69). The legacy of a research tradition in health care stemming largely from the tenets of logical positivism[1] has been particularly influential in framing discussions about the issues of appropriate and legitimate subject matter and methods for research.

Research in nursing, or in any other health area for that matter, should not draw on only one particular genre or type of research. Rather, "the research method should be consistent with the nature of the questions under investigation and the information gathered should be rigorously analysed" (Horsfall 1995, p 2). Hence, there is a place in nursing and health care for many different approaches to research. Such different approaches may open up previously overlooked or under-researched areas impinging on and influencing practice.

Indeed Dzurec (1989) asserts that "it is vital to nursing's ongoing development that openness to multiple paradigms be maintained" (p. 76), claiming that such multiple paradigms in the conduct of research are "an evolutionary necessity as well as a necessary stance for a responsible discipline" (p. 76).

A contemporary development in the evolution of nursing and health research has been the increasing prominence of the use of postmodern and poststructural approaches in researching the reality of health care. Even the most cursory of glances at the index of most contemporary nursing and health literature would reveal an ever-increasing number of books and articles exploring the potential of postmodern and poststructural thought for enabling new and different analyses of both nursing and health care practice.

Yet in most standard health and nursing *research* texts, postmodern and poststructural approaches do not get a mention, or if they do it is often only in passing in a relatively small section on qualitative techniques. Consequently, they remain somewhat marginalized and removed from the research reality of many health practitioners. Further, despite growing awareness of the potential that poststructural and postmodern approaches offer to health and nursing research and the concomitant advancement of health and nursing knowledge, these approaches are often either not well understood or not articulated theoretically—or both. Without a clear understanding of these approaches it is difficult to appreciate their application to research grounded in nursing/health care practice. In addition, examination of research reports about the use of these approaches reveals that there is often lack of detail about how one might actually research nursing/health using a poststructural or postmodern approach.

This book is written in response to this lack of clarity and to redress the absence of these approaches in standard nursing/health research methods and texts. Its intellectual contribution is to offer clearly delineated understandings of poststructural and postmodern approaches so that health professionals can use these approaches to inform their research. It is not to provide *"the"* definition of these terms, but to offer clear understandings in the sense of contextualising each approach from the points of view of where it comes from and what view of the world it offers. Once these foundational understandings have been established, this book will explore the implications of each approach for nursing and health care research.

In no way should this book be read as arguing that postmodern, poststructural—or any other form of thought for that matter—should assume the status of "truth," thereby excluding or constraining other ways of theorising and researching reality. Instead, the focus is on what postmodern and poststructural approaches can offer to analyses of health care. In this way these approaches become *"instruments* [italics added] *of analyses"* (Foucault 1980, p. 62), rather than *rigid sets of rules* for those analyses.

A brief glance at the table of contents will give you some idea of the way the book has been organized. Chapters 1, 2 and 3 explore the issue of what postmodern and poststructural approaches to research are and how they can be used to influence practice and inform us about aspects of the reality of health care. Each approach is discussed and examples are given to show how that approach has been used in health care research.

Having established a sound basis for the discussion to follow, the remaining chapters of the book explore the "how to" aspects of carrying out research using poststructural and postmodern approaches. It does so by discussing in depth actual examples of research that draw on these approaches. Put another way, these examples illustrate postmodern and poststructural research approaches in action. They discuss how to get started, how to write a proposal, how the project was conducted, how the data were analysed and what the outcomes of the research were—particularly with respect to tangible effects on practice. The use of examples of actual research as the vehicle for discussion ensures a relevant, accessible and practical focus for the discussion.

The book targets those interested in nursing and health-related research and those interested in learning how to go about using poststructural and postmodern research approaches in their practice context. In particular it targets:

–   final year undergraduate nursing or health science students undertaking research methods courses;

–   postgraduate nursing or health students in research methods classes and/or those who are preparing research proposals; and

–   nurses and other health care professionals working in practice settings who wish to learn about, and implement, poststructural and postmodern research approaches.

On a more philosophical level, the book should be of interest to all those who believe that nursing and health care does indeed matter and that research from a number of approaches, including those which are the focus of this text, is an integral and core activity in the evolution and development of nursing and health care knowledge and practice.

Having established what the book is about and the way it is organized, we will consider what is meant by postmodern and poststructural approaches.

TOWARDS AN UNDERSTANDING OF POSTMODERN AND POSTSTRUCTURAL APPROACHES

From the outset it must be stated that this discussion is necessarily introductory and exploratory, and that Chapters 2 and 3 will explore these approaches in greater depth.

Given the highly contestable nature of both the term *postmodern* and the term *poststructural*, it is not possible to arrive at *"a"* or *"the"* definition for either one. Therefore if you were hoping that I could provide you with a neat one- or two-line definition here you will be disappointed, and I make no apology for that! Working within the broad parameters of *postmodern* and *poststructural* are a number of writers each with particular emphases and consequent applications of postmodern and poststructural thought.

These approaches are thus more of "a set of intellectual propositions" (Bertens 1995, p. 9) or philosophical positions that privilege "no single authority, method or paradigm" (Denzin & Lincoln 1994, p. 15) than a single approach that can be clearly delineated. Postmodern and poststructural approaches are not research methods in themselves: rather they are ways of thinking about the world that shape the type of research that is done and the types of analyses that are utilized.

It is paradoxical that as the use of the terms *postmodern* and *poststructural* has increased in health-related literature, so has the ambiguity and lack of clarity with respect to both these approaches. Watson (1995), whilst recognising the potential of postmodern approaches for nursing analyses and even going so far as to suggest that nursing "must now yield to a postmodern approach" (p. 60), declares: "just exactly what is postmodernism is unknown and ambiguous at best" (p. 60). Indeed, Smart (1992) is moved to declare that *postmodern* and *poststructural* represent a "constellation of related terms all lacking in specificity" (p. 143) which fluctuates from one analyst to another! Such lack of specificity applies not only to the health literature but also to other disciplinary areas where these two approaches have also had a major impact on thought, on theorising and subsequently on research. For example, Agger (1992) asserts that "no cultural studies perspective is more ill-defined than the one(s) inspired by these two European traditions of thought" (p. 93).

Where, then, does this leave us? Is it the case that these terms are necessarily ambiguous and vague, unable to be defined? Or is it possible to attempt some clarity with respect to the debate about what these terms mean? Perhaps a good place to begin is to ask why there is such a lack of clarity. As we shall see throughout this book, much of the ambiguity arizes from the different ways in which these terms are used by writers. As Daniel (1995) points out, "there are so many different senses of postmodern (postmodernism or postmodernity) floating about today that no one description could respect all of the ways the term has been appropriated by theorists and commentators" (p. 256).

Part of the reason for this is that in many articles and books in the nursing/health literature, the understanding of these approaches in use is not clearly articulated. To "use" any approach requires an understanding of the origin of the thought implicit within the approach, what view of reality it promotes and conversely, what view it suppresses. In criticising the ambiguity associated with the terms *postmodern* and *poststructural*, Bloland (1995) noted that it is often assumed that "those who use the words also know the theory" (p. 522). Such an assumption does not always hold, and it is in the interests of removing the ambiguity that this book has been written.

Too often, writers assume shared understandings of what they are postulating with respect to postmodern or poststructural approaches. Of course this does not only apply to writers using postmodern or poststructural approaches. How often have you read research reports where the approach used, such as "grounded theory," "phenomenology," "thematic analysis" or even "qualitative design," is stated as a given and no further explanation is deemed necessary? Yet within grounded theory, phenomenology, thematic analysis and qualitative design there are a number of different perspectives each with its own emphasis and understandings. Simply stating the terms is not enough: the reason for choosing a particular approach to frame the analysis of a particular piece of research must be stated, as must the particular understanding of the approach being employed. This is important, especially with respect to postmodern and poststructural approaches, as these terms get "stretched in all directions across different debates, different disciplinary and discursive boundaries" (Hebdige 1988, p. 181).

Thus, what I am suggesting is that any research method or study which purports to draw on postmodern or poststructural approaches must clearly articulate the understanding of the approach that is being used.

As stated previously, given the highly contestable nature of both terms it is not possible to arrive at *"the"* definition for either one. Indeed, the very nature of the approaches themselves militates against this, as we shall see. However, *contestability of meaning* is not necessarily synonymous with *lack of clarity*. It is possible to explore the reasons for such contestability and to arrive at a stated position for any piece of work. Whilst not all may agree with such a stated position, at least it will be possible to determine what the position is. It is in this spirit that the following discussion is written.

All approaches and propositions considered as postmodern question the assumptions embedded within modernist thought. Indeed, postmodern thought has been described as a "crisis of confidence in the narratives of truth, science and progress that epitomized modernity" (Burman 1992, p. 98). The emphasis in modern theoretical analysis is on the big picture; that is, grand theories of social structure and action. Postmodern thought disavows the idea that human experience can be reduced to, and captured by, grand or totalising theories. Rather, postmodern thought emphasizes the plural nature of reality, the multiple positions from which it is possible to view any aspect of reality including health care and the partial nature of any representation of reality that arises from any form of writing/speaking that attempts to explore, describe or explain that reality.

Postmodern approaches can thus be described, at least in part, as a response to what has come to be viewed as a crisis in representation—a challenge to the view that it is possible to represent reality, speak for others, make truth claims and attain universal essential understandings. Postmodern approaches recognize the presence of multiple voices, multiple views and multiple methods when analysing any aspect of reality—including the reality of health care. Who and what is absent from representations of health care is thus of as much interest as who or what is *present*.

All of this challenges the notion of a rational and unified subject that is so central to modernist thought.

What is taken as being natural or normal, that is "a given" or "truth," is open to question and challenge in postmodern approaches. This includes the everyday practice setting of the health practitioner. For example, instead of seeking to describe and understand how that practice setting functions, postmodern approaches allow for the possibility of exploring how the practice setting came to be constructed in the way that it is. What are the assumptions and understandings of health care practice taken that are for granted which have shaped the way practice settings operate? Whose assumptions and understandings are they, and why are other views excluded or marginalized?

A working definition, based on and clarifying the preceding discussion, of postmodern approaches is that offered by Best and Kellner (1991) It states that postmodern approaches reject "modern assumptions of social coherence and notions of causality in favour of multiplicity, plurality, fragmentation, and indeterminacy" (p. 4). As mentioned previously, Chapter 2 will explore in more detail both postmodern thought and its applicability to research in the health care arena.

Well then, what of poststructural approaches? What is a working definition for these approaches? Poststructural approaches have much in common with postmodern approaches: in fact some writers have used the terms interchangeably. Like postmodern approaches, poststructuralist approaches value plurality, fragmentation and multi-vocality. However they differ from postmodern approaches in terms of their focus and emphasis.

Poststructural approaches tend to focus on the exploration and analysis of *texts* where texts refer to representations of reality. In poststructuralist approaches, texts for analysis may include, for example, patient case notes and media representations of health and illness. The representation of aspects of health care and attendant health care practices, whether spoken, acted or written texts, is the focus of a poststructural analysis. Squier (1993) neatly encapsulates both what such research is about and a working understanding of poststructural approaches when she writes that the task of poststructural research approaches is to "investigate the meaning of particular representations: to understand how they came to be as they are, and what they communicate about their specific cultural and historical contexts" (p. 30).

Like postmodern approaches, poststructural approaches themselves are plural; that is, having more than one fixed meaning. Nevertheless poststructural approaches all "share certain fundamental assumptions about language, meaning and subjectivity" (Weedon 1987, p. 19). In a poststructural approach language itself is explored in terms of the role that it plays in both conveying and constructing understandings about, and representations of, reality.

This is almost where we will leave our discussion of poststructural approaches. This introductory discussion is picked up on and developed greatly in Chapter 3 which explores poststructural thought and how it can be applied to health care practices in detail.

A final word is necessary, however, before we leave this introduction to postmodern and poststructural approaches. Although for the purposes of convenience I have divided the structure of the book into individual chapters about postmodern approaches and poststructural approaches, this is not to imply that such a neat division is without problems. I have already stated that these approaches have much ground in common: valuing plurality of thought and perspective and challenging aspects of reality taken for granted, including the health care realm. As Agger (1992) declares about these approaches, "at some level, they are so inextricably linked as to make simplistic differentiations impossible or undesirable" (p. 109). Indeed, Daniel (1995) argues that poststructuralism, like critical theory and deconstruction, needs to be "situated within a broadly postmodern context" (p. 257). Likewise Best and Kellner (1991, p. 25) argue that poststructuralism forms part of "the matrix of postmodern theory" and thus a subset of a broader approach.

Consequently it is not possible to clearly separate postmodernism from poststructuralism. This is evident from the way in which various theorists are described as "poststructural" by some and "postmodern" by others. For example, whilst Derrida is usually classified as poststructural (although he does not identify himself as such), Foucault (who also resisted categorising himself) has been described as both poststructuralist and postmodern. Like these two prominent theorists, postmodern and poststructural approaches resist being placed into neat, clearly delineated categories. However, while there are many similarities between these two approaches, as we have seen, each does have its own specific emphases (Daniel 1995) and levels of focus. We will explore this further in Chapters 2 and 3.

CAN POSTMODERN AND POSTSTRUCTURALIST APPROACHES INFLUENCE PRACTICE OR ARE THEY MERELY ESOTERIC?

We have briefly established the organisation of the book and the focus of the discussion and begun to explore what is meant by postmodern and poststructural approaches to research. This section now considers an issue that will be a key thread running throughout the discussion in the entire book. It pertains to the question of whether or not postmodern and poststructural approaches are able to inform the practical reality of the health care setting.

Some critics would claim that these approaches are merely esoteric and inward looking, unable to make any contribution to health care practice at all. Put another way, drawing on Popper's (1976) examination of critical theory, it can be asked whether such approaches are anything more than trivialities in high-sounding language. If that is so, then we should abandon our discussion at this point, for what is the value of an approach to research in health care, the product of which cannot contribute to improvement and development in health care practice? The answer, obviously, is very little value, if any.

There are many critiques that discuss the seeming inability of studies using postmodern and poststructural approaches to influence the everyday reality of health care practice. I wish to cite one example drawn from the nursing literature. In so doing, my intention is to provide an introduction to such critiques, not to offer an overview or aggregation of critics and their various stances. Further, neither is it my intention to somehow privilege the critique offered in the example chosen above other critics and/or critiques. What is my intention is to set the parameters for what is to follow in the book by introducing readers to one example of the type of critique that is often levelled at postmodern and poststructural approaches to research. More extensive discussion of the limitations and critiques of each of the approaches will be offered in Chapters 2 and 3.

Kermode and Brown (1996) typify critics who suggest that postmodern and poststructuralist approaches, in terms of their ability to influence practice in the health context, are of little value. In an attack on postmodernism and its increasing prominence in the nursing literature they assert:

> postmodernism is at best a distraction, and at worst, an epistemological hoax concocted by white bourgeois patriarchy to divert women and other oppressed groups from participating in the Enlightenment project, while the real narrative rolls on relentlessly—capitalism, patriarchy and power. (p. 380)

Indeed, they go on to suggest that because "postmodernist constructions of knowledge are necessarily local, contextual and readily contestable, their social significance is minuscule" (p. 383). Some of the questions (and there are probably many more) that immediately arise from Kermode and Brown's analysis are as follows:

– Postmodernism is "at best a distraction" from *what*?

– Is this to suggest that white, bourgeois[2] patriarchy[3] have participated in some kind of conspiracy designed to deliberately set out to ensnare unsuspecting groups such as women, in what can only ever be an "alternate" approach given the implied and assumed pre-eminence of the Enlightenment[4] project underpinned by the tenets of scientific rationality?

– Who or what determines what the "real" narrative is, and how do they know? and *very* importantly:

– Is the "social significance" of "local, contextual and contestable" knowledge necessarily minuscule?

Thus what Kermode and Brown *don't* say is just as important as what they *do*. Like researchers using postmodern perspectives, Kermode and Brown approach their research, their critique of other theories and their judgments about the value (or lack of it) of certain types of research from a particular world view or what Gouldner (1971) terms "background assumptions." This highlights Chia's (1996) assertion of an "increasing realisation that the researcher/theorist [critic] plays an active role in constructing the very reality he/she is attempting to investigate" (p. 42).

The position from which commentators take up their critique of postmodern and poststructural approaches is an important issue, but it is often ignored especially with respect to discussions about the value of these approaches in terms of their ability to influence or change practice. Mullhall (1995) neatly encapsulates the central point I am making when she states that "the attachment to traditional and already accepted concepts and paradigms may also overwhelm new evidence presenting a different view....certain people define phenomena in certain ways, and once defined there is considerable resistance to change" (p. 580). This point becomes especially apparent if the politics of research funding is considered.

The fact is that despite recognition of the possibilities afforded by multiple perspectives and approaches to research in nursing and health care, not all approaches within the research enterprise are afforded equal credibility and standing. Often such legitimacy is conferred by certain groups who have a certain view about what constitutes "valid" research and "valid" research methods. One such group may be those who fund research. As Gilbert (1995) posits, "the present forms of truth and rationality determine the issues acceptable for research monies and for publication" (p. 869).

In the climate of economic rationalism that pervades contemporary western society, cost and cost benefits have become a prime focus for evaluating the value of a certain health care procedure or organisation. The same is true for research. This is particularly so as universities are increasingly urged to "pay their way," so that funding for research rather than the quality of the research itself often becomes the hallmark of success. "Pressure is therefore exerted on academics to tailor their work in order to meet the requirements of funders" (Porter 1997, p. 655). The power and influence of funding bodies to determine both research priorities and ways in which that research should be carried out have been steadily increasing in this climate. One way this power and influence is manifested is in the funding of only certain types of research.

One key consideration for many funding bodies is the immediacy of the effects of the recommendations of the research undertaken. In such a view, research must be able to immediately and directly affect practice by enabling the swift implementation of recommendations. However as Porter (1997) points out:

> What this approach misses out is recognition of the importance of the "basic" research upon which more applied and instrumental research is founded. While this research may have a less immediate impact upon practice, it is nonetheless an essential factor in the development of nursing. (p. 656)

What we are really talking about here is the nature of the research product or, to use a term that is achieving much prominence in contemporary research rhetoric, the "deliverable(s)." Research deliverables are increasingly being defined as recommendations, strategies and models for best practice and/or cost efficiency in health service delivery. Whilst there is no doubt that such deliverables can have a positive impact on the content and delivery of care, and thus should be a focus of health based research, they should not be the *only* focus. There is room for other research approaches and outcomes that can inform understandings of practice itself. If we are only interested in improving what is, it may well be that we will never explore what might be.

Postmodern and poststructural research approaches may not be able to produce cost-benefit analysis on their own, but they may be able to provide the basis for conceptualising practice in new or different ways which then can be analysed in further studies (or even in another part of the same multifaceted study). Thus, although research from these approaches may be "once removed" in terms of how immediate the applicability of the findings are, this type of research can influence and inform basic understandings in health care delivery.

To illustrate this point, I will briefly refer to some of the outcomes of a research project I recently completed. The study was called "Constructing Toxic Shock Syndrome: Selected Australian Print-Based Media Representations of Toxic Shock Syndrome from 1979-1995." This research explored the discursive (see Chapter 2) construction of a relatively new health phenomenon, Toxic Shock Syndrome (TSS) by Australian print-based media. In so doing, it aimed to provide insights into ways print-based texts represent health issues, thereby influencing attitudes towards health, towards those with certain illnesses and towards health care practices. Thus, in the section of the proposal asking for direct applications of research results, I was able to make the following points. The study would:

– provide better understanding of the way in which "popular" magazines (a largely neglected research focus) and newspapers frame and represent health issues and risk with respect to TSS, and

– explore ways in which these print-based media might better communicate understandings of health and health risks.

I then went on to point out that once such representation is analysed and its effects are better understood, it will be possible to design relevant health promotion strategies and information packages pertaining to TSS, the use of tampons, and other related health issues for both consumers and health professionals.

Clearly this study provides what Porter (1997) has termed "basic" research upon which can be founded more applied and instrumental research on delivering a clearly defined product for a specific goal. The understandings provided by this study have the potential to inform and influence the delivery of health care and attendant health care practices. Indeed, even strident critics such as Kermode and Brown (1996) are grudgingly forced to concede that "as methods and procedures for gathering and interpreting data, postmodernist approaches may produce a useful starting point in some areas" (p. 383).

All of this is to recognize that the criticism that is often leveled at postmodern, poststructural and other research approaches about their apparent inability to contribute to practice and health care delivery may well be more a political criticism than a methodological one. It is a criticism premised on a certain understanding of what a research deliverable or product is, or should be, particularly in terms of its perceived immediate instrumental applicability.

Much of this understanding is derived from an increasingly pervasive discourse of economic rationalism in the health care sector. Porter (1997) captures this neatly when he asserts that "in short there is an economic disincentive...to fund research that may have generalized long-term effects, but which is unlikely to deliver immediate, locally applicable results" (p. 656).

It is most important to appreciate that postmodern and poststructural research approaches can and do influence practice and contribute to understandings of health care delivery. Perhaps what they do not do is reach findings and come up with conclusions in a way that suits the interests of certain powerful groups. This includes some funding bodies which have their own political agenda and for which the allocation of research funding for certain types of projects and not others may be a way of maintaining their own power and world view (Dzurec 1989).

Therefore, far from accepting Kermode and Brown's (1996) polemic assertion that "the attractions of postmodernism are self-defeating for an occupation such as nursing" (p. 375), the rest of this book will demonstrate that it is self-defeating for occupations such as nursing, *not* to pursue postmodern and poststructural approaches to research.

To ignore such approaches is to forfeit the potential for nursing and health research to evolve and develop multiple research approaches from which to explore the reality of health care provision. It is to "sell-out" to the agendas of others—agendas which are often more political than interested in the worth of particular methodological approaches.

From all of this arises the question of whether the encroachment in American universities of what Nisbet (1971) terms "academic entrepreneurs, engaged in the sale of knowledge designed for instrumental use by those who bought it" (p. 239) and which results in "the degradation of the academic values that had animated universities since their foundation" (p. 239) could become true of research in the nursing/health sphere if *only* instrumental ends are pursued. That is what would be truly self-defeating for occupations such as nursing, for as Street (1997) asserts:

> Nurses need to be encouraged and assisted to take time to think deeply about nursing. We are all under pressure: pressure that seduces us to respond and react, rather than to think and act. Yet when thinking is valued and fostered, action can be effective and efficient. (p. 79)

Postmodern and poststructural approaches offer one way of thinking deeply about nursing and health care. Practical, specific and concrete research outcomes are needed in practice-based disciplines such as nursing, but so are thoughtful practitioners who can influence and change practice. The two need not be mutually exclusive.

WHAT IS TO FOLLOW

This chapter has set the parameters for the way in which this book is organized, what it aims to achieve and the major points that form the focus of the discussion to follow. These points are amplified in Chapters 2 and 3.

Chapter 2 is specifically concerned with *postmodern* thought. It provides an overview of this type of thought and explores why it is often viewed as ambiguous and hard to define. Rather than providing "the" definition of postmodernism, the chapter situates postmodernism theoretically, adds depth to a working definition of a postmodern approach and considers the work of one of the most influential theorists whose work has been associated with this perspective— Michel Foucault. Examples of how researchers have used Foucauldian analysis to inform our understandings of aspects of health care are provided and discussed. In particular, Foucault's notion of *discourse* is explored.

Chapter 3 turns the reader's attention to *poststructural* thought. A key point is made at the outset (one on which we have already touched briefly in this chapter), namely that *poststructural* and *postmodern* are in many ways closely related terms and are often used synonymously. However, our exploration reveals that poststructural analyses are often concerned with an analysis of texts that represent aspects of reality. Discourse analysis as a method/approach for analysing texts is discussed with particular reference to a study of case notes by Cheek and Rudge (1994b; 1994e).

The usefulness of Parker's (1992) four phases or stages for discourse analysis is explored by juxtaposing the stages identified by Parker and the analysis that occurred in a research project on the way nurses are represented with respect to the quality administration of medications. The final section of the chapter briefly considers the work of Derrida and the potential afforded by deconstructive approaches to analyses of health care and health care delivery.

The remaining chapters of the book are more focused on the "how to" aspects of employing postmodern and poststructural approaches in nursing and health care research. Specifically, Chapter 4 explores postmodern and poststructural research approaches in terms of writing a research proposal drawing on these approaches. Areas explored include:

–   writing for a particular audience;
–   defining the issue/question of what constitutes a topic that can be researched;
–   using the literature to help define the research issue/question;
–   using the theoretical perspective drawn upon to inform the method; and
–   specifying practical outcomes and benefits of the research in terms of health care practice.

The discussion is based around a proposal I wrote for a research project I have successfully completed and which is mentioned previously in this chapter ("Constructing Toxic Shock Syndrome: Selected Australian print-based media representations of Toxic Shock Syndrome from 1979-1995"). The discussion is thus grounded in the reality of actual research. Excerpts from the proposal are used to illustrate the points and the reasons why certain decisions were made are discussed. Three levels of analysis and discussion operate throughout this chapter: the actual content of the proposal; meeting the requirements of the funding body or other audience for whom the proposal is written; and the research proposal itself as an example of text and of the unwritten rules and assumptions that shape its form and content.

Chapter 5 continues to use the study explored in Chapter 4 as the main vehicle for discussion. It considers the questions of what type of data might be collected and how such data might be analysed. Excerpts of data will be cited and the analysis process described. In this chapter, the reader is encouraged to participate in analysing the examples given and to write their reactions to the discussion as it unfolds. These jottings will prove invaluable to the development of an understanding of these approaches by the reader, thereby promoting an active reader who can engage with the material being presented.

Chapter 6, the concluding chapter, serves two purposes. The first is to offer a brief summary of the material covered in the book and to emphasize the contribution to understandings of nursing and health care practice that poststructural and postmodern approaches to research can offer. It is designed to encourage readers to pursue their own research interests.

The discussion will also highlight further sources of information for the researcher working alone or wanting to learn more about these approaches to research and to understanding the world. The second purpose of this chapter is to emphasize both the possibilities and pitfalls of this type of research for understanding nursing and health care. The book concludes by emphasising the importance of research to the development of nursing knowledge.

The contribution of this book to the field of nursing/health research is twofold. Firstly, it provides a clear overview of poststructural and postmodern approaches, situating them with respect to their philosophical and social science research traditions and portraying both the strengths and limitations of these perspectives. Secondly, it provides a practical discussion of how to put into operation research that draws on postmodern and poststructural approaches. This is done using examples of actual research, and discusses very basic, practical information. The book therefore becomes a "critical friend" to the reader, discussing the research process at each stage, the reasons for decisions, the problems encountered and the outcome or product of the research.

FURTHER READINGS

Agger, B. (1991). Critical theory, post structuralism, post modernism: Their sociological relevance. *Annual Review of Sociology, 17*, 105-131.

Here Agger provides a good working definition of critical theory, poststructural and postmodern thought and their methodological implications for research and application to sociology. The article also introduces the work of a number of central theorists including Derrida and Foucault and contains excellent discussions of deconstruction and of what constitutes text.

Dzurec, L. (1989). The necessity for and evolution of multiple paradigms for nursing research: A poststructuralist perspective. *Advances in Nursing Science, 11*(4), 69-77.

Dzurec introduces Foucault's concept of power and knowledge and uses this to critique two paradigms in nursing research—positivism and phenomenology. The author points to the dominance of positivist "scientific" methods and highlights the power relations evident within that dominance. She argues that nursing needs to develop multiple paradigms and research methods.

Horsfall, J. (1995). Madness in our methods: Nursing research and epistemology. *Nursing Inquiry, 2*, 2-9.

Horsfall criticizes positivist scientific methods as being inappropriate and limiting to nursing. Central to her criticism is the separation of the researcher from the subjects of research. She sees this as reductive; as ignoring the complexities of the social lives of the subjects; as ignoring the power relations between subject and researcher; and as leading to a lack of empathy for, and understanding of, subject positions.

Kermode, S. & Brown, C. (1996). The postmodern hoax and its effects on nursing. *International Journal of Nursing Studies, 33*(4), 375-384.

This article criticizes postmodern thought on the grounds that it ignores grand narratives and major social divisions such as class and gender, does not have a moral prescription for action and thereby reinforces the status quo. The authors argue that this is detrimental to nursing as it ignores the social conditions that lead to the oppression of nurses and to differing health outcomes across class, gender and race lines. They also see it as furthering medical power because it does not provide a critique of the status quo.

Mitchell, D. (1996). Postmodernism, health and illness. *Journal of Advanced Nursing, 23*, 201-2021a5.

Mitchell introduces a number of key postmodern concepts and argues for their application to nursing research. The author uses Foucauldian theory to examine the dominance and legitimacy of scientific/medical knowledge, arguing that it governs the research through the imposition on it of power relations and that medical/scientific knowledge is but one discourse among many possible ways of viewing the body of research.

NOTES

1. Positivism is identified with a "conviction that [nursing health] can be scientific in the same way as, say, physics, a marked preference for measurement and quantification, and a tendency towards social structural explanations as distinct from those which refer to human intentions and motives" (Abercrombie, Hill & Turner 1988, p. 190).

2. Bourgeoisie (plural of bourgeois). Bourgeois "This term is used loosely to describe either the middle or ruling classes in capitalist society" (Abercrombie et al. 1988, p. 22).

3. "This concept is used to describe the dominance of men over women, a dominance which appears in several quite different kinds of society" (Abercrombie et al. 1988, p.181).

4. The Enlightenment is a way of thinking arising from the 17th Century Scientific Revolution. The central feature of the Enlightenment is a belief that all aspects of nature, including human nature and society, are regulated by universal natural laws that can be uncovered through the application of "scientific methods of observation and deduction" (Hampson 1993, p. 195). The individual is seen as rational and self-interested.

Chapter 2

Situating Postmodern Thought

WHAT THIS CHAPTER IS ABOUT

This chapter begins by exploring what postmodern thought is. Rather than just providing a definition (which as we shall see is a difficult task in itself) the discussion seeks to contextualize the understanding of postmodern thought by giving a sense of where such thought has come from and to what it might be considered a reaction. Having done so, the discussion draws out common threads within postmodern thought and arrives at a "working understanding" of a postmodern approach that will be used throughout the book.

The chapter then turns to consider the work of Michel Foucault, one of the most influential theorists associated with postmodern theory. As we shall see, Foucault resisted the location of his work into any neat theoretical category. Nevertheless, many of his analyses are in keeping with postmodern thought, and this section of the chapter focuses on how Foucauldian perspectives can be used to explore and analyze aspects of contemporary health practice. Foucault's concept of discourse is especially useful in this respect.

Having examined some of the central theses of Foucault's argument, the discussion turns to look at how Nettleton (1991) used the concept of governmentality to research the discourses and practices surrounding the mouth and teeth and how such discursive frames shape contemporary understandings and practices in dental health care. We then return to Foucault's concept of the panoptic gaze as central to contemporary conceptualizations of the clinic and attendant health care practices.

The final section of the chapter explores what research from a postmodern approach might actually look at and what it might involve. Examples of research using this approach are discussed.

WHAT IS POSTMODERN THOUGHT?

Postmodern thought has gained increasing import and interest in many disciplinary fields since World War II. Indeed, in the past two decades postmodern debates have dominated many fields of study throughout the world (Best & Kellner 1991). Initially postmodern thought influenced predominantly the fields of art and architecture; but contemporary writings reveal its spread to philosophy and literary studies in the 1950s and 1960s, and in the 1970s, 1980s and 1990s into virtually all fields of culture and study including nursing and health care.

Postmodern thought has been strongly influenced by French theorists such as Foucault, Lyotard, Baudrillard and Derrida, although, as stated in chapter 1, many of these theorists reject the placement of their work into any particular category—including that of postmodernism. Best and Kellner in their "Postmodern Theory: Critical Interrogations" (1991) provide a succinct yet comprehensive overview of what they term the archaeology of the postmodern, and if you want to read more about the influence of particular theorists and schools of thought on the development of understandings of the postmodern this is an excellent place to start.

Postmodern thought represents an unstable concept (Bauman 1992) that is hard to define in that it does not represent a unified position or a coherent school of thought. Rather, as Best and Kellner (1991) point out, "one is struck by the diversities between theories often lumped together as 'postmodern' and the plurality—often conflictual—of postmodern positions" (p. 2). For example, there is diversity of thought as to what the prefix post refers to in the term postmodern. Some writers view the prefix as a "periodizing concept whose function is to correlate the emergence of new features in culture" (Sarup 1989, p. 131) where post refers to the next step in the historical development of ideas and cultural features in contemporary Western society. In this sense postmodernism is post in that it follows and succeeds the modern era. Others view the prefix post as signifying "an active rupture (coupure) with what preceded it" (Best & Kellner 1991, p. 29)—namely modernity and modern thought.

This is not to suggest, however, that there is nothing in common among those positions and approaches termed postmodern. All postmodern approaches emerge from a critique of the assumptions that underpin modernist thought. Indeed Bauman (1992) declares that it is the dismantling of the artifice of modernity, and all that that artifice is premised on, that is the focus of postmodern thought. For example, postmodern thought problematizes modernist understandings of history as having a definite direction which is ultimately progressive, the desire for universal and generalizable categories of explanation, a belief in reason as the basis for action and a belief that "the nation state could coordinate and advance such developments for the whole society and thereby constitute society itself" (Parton 1994, p. 101).

Thus postmodern thought discards the organic notion of all parts of society working together in an orderly way, and in so doing it rejects "modern assumptions of social coherence and notions of causality in favour of multiplicity, plurality, fragmentation, and indeterminacy" (Best & Kellner 1991, p. 4).So, for example, postmodern thought challenges the very persuasive metaphor of the health care system as a system where all components and players work together for a common good. It also problematizes the notion of "advances" and "progress" in health care both in terms of what actually constitutes progress and advances, and concomitantly, whether developments and change in the health care system are necessarily progressive.

Postmodern thought thus rejects grand theories which aim to offer totalizing descriptions and explanations of both history and social structures. Lyotard (1984), a French postmodern writer, in his foundational work "The Postmodern Condition: A Report on Knowledge," encapsulates his understanding of postmodern thought in the following statement: "Simplifying to the extreme, I define postmodern as incredulity towards metanarratives" (p. xxiv). By metanarratives, Lyotard is referring to conceptual and theoretical schema that attempt to link and represent all aspects of reality coherently in a way that is supposedly consistent and true. The metanarrative embodies "the supposedly transcendent and universal truths that underpin western civilization and that function to give the civilization objective legitimation" (Bertens 1995, p. 124).

Indeed, incoherence rather than the notion of a coherent society is one of, if not the, distinctive feature of postmodern thought (Bauman 1992). Agger (1992) captures this idea neatly when he states that postmodernism "is a theory of cultural, intellectual and societal discontinuity that rejects the linearism of Enlightenment notions of progress" (p. 93). Rather than seeking universal and essential truths, postmodern thought recognizes the existence of multiple perspectives, assuming instead plurality of understandings for any aspect of social reality. Consequently:

> if we are entering a post-modern age, then one of its most distinctive characteristics is a loss of rational and social coherence in favour of cultural images and social forms and identities marked by fragmentation, multiplicity, plurality and indeterminacy. (Thompson 1992, p. 223)

The recognition of reality as comprised of multiple voices, views and representations challenges the idea of a rational and unified subject that is at the core of modernist tenets. Rather, postmodern thought suggests a subject that is "socially and linguistically decentred and fragmented" (Best & Kellner 1991, p. 5). Thus, postmodern approaches:

> in their own way … all seek to transcend what they see as the self-imposed limitations of modernism, which in its search for autonomy and purity or for timeless, representational, truth has subjected experience to unacceptable intellectualizations and reductions. (Bertens 1995, p. 5)

Yet this is not to suggest that postmodern thought attacks all reason and discounts rationality in order to glorify irrationality (Daniel 1995). Rather, it is to highlight the constructed nature of what have often become "truths" and taken-for-granted aspects of our reality. This includes practices and procedures in the health domain. It is important to recognize that:

> because postmodernity undermines the fascination of truth itself, it does not offer itself as the truth. Instead...it is an invitation to consider how things would be different if we were to adopt such beliefs, an invitation to imagine what would happen if we were to think this or that way. (Daniel 1995, p. 266)

Thus, postmodern thought is enabling in that it encourages us to think about reality in a reflexive way. Such reflexivity unmasks "complex political/ideological agendas hidden in our writing [and practice]. Truth claims are less easily validated now; desires to speak 'for' others are suspect" (Richardson 1994, p. 523). Thus, as much as postmodern thought is "undetermined" it is also "undetermining" in that it serves to, "weaken... the constraining impact of the past and effectively prevent... colonization of the future" (Bauman 1992, p. 190). However it is important to note at this point that because postmodern thought seems to ensure that every point of view is heard and that none be privileged above others, postmodern thought has been challenged by some critics as being amoral.

Where does all this leave us? First, it is apparent that postmodern thought rejects the concept of an ever onward and upward progress as epitomized by the project of modernity. Postmodern thought disavows the idea that human experience can be reduced to and captured by grand or totalizing theories, the metanarratives of which Lyotard was so critical. Rather, postmodern thought emphasizes that reality is plural and that there are multiple positions from which it is possible to view any aspect of reality. This applies to the often taken-for-granted reality of nursing and health care. Any writing/speaking done about nursing or health care is an attempt to explore that reality. It will and can only ever be a partial analysis, in that it draws on only one of a number of possible positions from which to view the reality in question.

This has implications for health/nursing research and researchers. If reality is made up of multiple voices, and if there are multiple positions from which to view that reality, then it follows that no single representation of health care or nursing practice can hope to capture the "truth" about that care or practice. Rather, any representation of health/nursing offers one of a number of possibilities for analyzing the reality in question. This includes the methods, and even the questions, that researchers choose to employ in any study of aspects of health care reality:

> Researchers should become more aware of how their own positions and interests are imposed at all stages of the research process—from the questions they ask to those they ignore, from whom they study to whom they ignore, from problem formation to analysis, representation and writing. (Hertz 1996, p. 5)

Thus, researchers working within the frame of postmodern thought need to be aware of the role that such thought plays in framing the parameters of the study, the methods employed to obtain "data," the analyses that are then done and the conclusions that are reached. What (or who) is absent, or not stated, in any research undertaken is of as much importance as what (or who) is present or stated. Postmodern thought argues that "every knowledge is contextualized by its historical and cultural nature" (Agger 1991, p. 117). This requires researchers to expose rather than conceal (for instance, behind methodological frames) "their own investment in a particular view of the world" (Agger 1991, p. 117). As Fox (1991) declares, "postmodernism requires of its practitioners that they recognize the personal values and commitments immanent in their own analyses" (p. 711), including the very research questions they ask and the methods they employ to seek answers to those questions.

In summary, there is no neat, clearly delineated definition of postmodern thought. However, the following excerpt from Parton (1994) encapsulates where our discussion has led us in terms of establishing working understandings of such thought:

> While diverse, there are clearly important points of connection between different (post) modern theorists in their discussions of the decentring of the subject, the rejection of "grand narratives," the espousal of "local narratives"... the dread of totalising discourses leading to totalitarianism... political pluralism and recovery of the "other" (p.109).

This is as close as we will come to a "perfect" definition of postmodern thought. It is important to remember that postmodernism is a way of thinking about reality just as any theoretical perspective is. Indeed, one of postmodernism's great contributions to nursing and health care analyses is to highlight how theory itself, along with the research methods and approaches associated or congruent with any particular theoretical orientation, frames our understandings of what is appropriate subject matter to study in the first place. The unsettling effect of postmodern thought on what we may have come to take for granted in health practice realms is one of its greatest contributions—offering possibilities for bringing about change and allowing "other" voices and perspectives to surface.

Best and Kellner (1991) provide us with a useful framework to use when reading and critiquing work that draws on postmodern thought. Although they use this framework in their book for exploring the work of various postmodern theorists, equally it can be used to explore writing in the health and nursing arena that uses postmodern approaches. For each postmodern theorist they examine how that theorist:

> (1) characterize[s] and criticize[s] modernity and its discourses; (2) postulate[s] a break with modernity and modern theory; (3) produce[s] alternative postmodern theories, positions, or perspectives; (4) create[s], or fail[s] to create, a theory of postmodernity; and (5) provide[s], or fail[s] to develop a new postmodern politics adequate to the supposed postmodern situation (p. 32).

While not suggesting that every analysis or article in the health or nursing sphere using a postmodern approach should, or indeed could, cover all of these points, they nevertheless provide a useful frame to interrogate the discussion for the underlying premises regarding postmodern thought on which the analysis in question is founded.

Having established a working understanding of postmodern thought and a possible way of exploring the type of thought underpinning analyses using postmodern approaches, this chapter considers the work of one of the most influential theorists associated with postmodern theory—Michel Foucault.

THE WORK OF MICHEL FOUCAULT

One theorist whose work has been consistently associated with postmodern perspectives is the French social theorist Michel Foucault. However, Foucault himself resisted the placement of his work in any particular theoretical category, describing it instead as a "history of the present" (Foucault 1977, p. 31). Further, Foucault's work is very difficult to categorize in a traditional disciplinary sense. As Foster (1985) asks, "is the work of Michel Foucault...to be called philosophy, history, social theory or political science?" (p. x). Such difficulty stems, at least in part, from the fact that Foucauldian analyses, in keeping with postmodern analyses, are "'in between' and 'across' established boundaries of knowledge" (Dean 1994, p. 13). Despite such uncertainty in explicitly labeling or categorizing Foucault's work, an exploration of aspects of his work will illuminate some of the understandings of postmodern posited previously.

Discourse

We will begin the exploration of Foucault's work by focusing on his problematization of knowledge. Foucault challenges notions which hold that knowledge is objective and value-free, inevitably progressive, and universal. He argues instead that knowledge is inextricably bound to power. In so doing, he attacks "great systems, good theories and vital truths" (Burrell 1998 p.223) and argued that "there is no unity of history, no unity of the subject, no sense of progress, no acceptance of the History of Ideas" (Burrell 1988, p 229). Foucault explores the knowledge/power link through the concept of discourse. For Foucault "discourse" refers to ways of thinking and speaking about aspects of reality:

> A discourse provides a set of possible statements about a given area, and organizes and gives structure to the manner in which a particular topic, object, process is to be talked about (Kress 1985, p. 7).

Thus, a discourse consists of a set of common assumptions which, although they may be so taken for granted as to be invisible, provide the basis for conscious knowledge.

Discourses create discursive frameworks which order reality in a certain way. They both enable and constrain the production of knowledge in that they allow for certain ways of thinking about reality whilst excluding others. In this way they determine who can speak, when, and with what authority, and conversely, who can not (Ball 1990). In analyzing the effect of such discursive frames, Foucault asks, "what rules permit certain statements to be made; what rules order these statements; what rules permit us to identify some statements as true and some false; what rules allow for construction of a map, model, or classificatory system" (Philp 1985, p. 69)?

It is important to recognize that at any point in time there are a number of possible discursive frames for thinking, writing and speaking about aspects of reality. However, not all discourses are afforded equal presence or, therefore, equal authority. At any time in history certain discourses will operate in such a way as to marginalize or even exclude others. Romanyshyn (1989), for example, uses understandings of the dead body to illustrate how certain ways of thinking can operate at various points in history to marginalize or exclude others. He identifies Vesalius as the founder of modern anatomy in 1543, and examines the way in which the discursive framework constituting understandings of anatomy led to different ways of viewing the same object—the human corpse/dead body. The study of anatomy led to new and different ways of knowing about and understanding the human body:

> Before Vesalius the non-living body was a dead body. Dead bodies are buried with rituals of remembrance. After Vesalius the dead body became a corpse. Corpses are designed to be opened for inspection. They are invented so that the inside can be instructive about the outside. (Romanyshyn 1989, pp. 16-17)

Knowledge of anatomy, premised on scientific/medical discourse, has assumed dominance in contemporary understandings of health and health care. It has had the effect of marginalizing, or relegating to the position of "other" alternate understandings of the human body such as spiritual ones which at other times in history had been dominant.

Which discursive frame is afforded presence at any time is a consequence of the effect of power relations. "Discourses represent political interests and in consequence are constantly vying for status or power" (Weedon 1987, p. 41). Indeed Foucault (1984) declares: "Discourse is the power which is to be seized" (p. 110). In Foucault's analysis, power is thus a productive concept: it is not simply repressive. It is the operation of webs of power that enables certain knowledge to be produced and "known."

Paradoxically, such power also constrains what it is possible to know in certain situations. The human body itself, as object of scientific/medical scrutiny is both constructed by, and in turn assists in the construction of, scientific/medical discourse—"in short, the human body is both target and effect of medical practice" (Armstrong ,1985, p. 111).

Knowledge from within one discourse can be used to *exclude* knowledge from other discourses. The fact that some discourses (in this case, scientific/medical understandings of the body) gain prominence over others is the result of socio-historical influences operating upon them (Cheek & Rudge 1994d). They achieve "truth" status where truth "is an effect of the rules of a discourse" (Cheek & Rudge 1993, p. 275).

In contemporary health care the truth status of medical/scientific discursive frames has shaped dominant taken-for-granted understandings of what is appropriate and authoritative practice. The ability and right of certain groups of health professions rather than others to speak authoritatively about health and illness is premised on the authority of the scientific/medical discourse from which their expertise is both derived and in turn legitimated. As Turner (1987) puts it:

> The power of the [medical] profession... depends, at least in part, on the ability to make claims successfully about the scientific value of their work and the way in which their professional knowledge is grounded in precise, accurate and reliable scientific information. (p. 217)

This power also depends on the ability to exclude or marginalize other ways of thinking about health care and health care practice, often relegating these other knowledges to the realm of the "alternative" health care practices, rather than the mainframe of authoritative contemporary health care. As Davies (1989) notes:

> If we see society as being constantly created through discursive practices then it is possible to see the power of those practices, not only to create and sustain the social world but also to see how we can change that world through a refusal of certain discourses and the generation of new ones. (p. xi)

For example, understandings of nurses and nursing are shaped by the context and understandings within which nurses and nursing operate. Such understandings frame the ways nurses view themselves and how they are viewed by others. Often nursing is positioned and portrayed with respect to its relation to scientific/medical discourse rather than in terms of nursing discourse. Consequently we find that nurses themselves have spent considerable time focusing on the science of nursing, often to the exclusion of the art of nursing (Johnson 1994). How nurses and nursing are portrayed, both by themselves and by others, is to a large extent the result of powers and practices that operate to position nursing in one way rather than another.

The aspects of nursing that are given prominence and the aspects that are absent reveal much about both ways of thinking about nursing and nurses embedded within certain understandings of health and health care practice. Put another way, it exposes the dominant discursive frames shaping nursing and nurses at any point in time.

Thus as I have suggested elsewhere, "the task is not to look for *real* and authentic representations of nursing, but rather to look for the speaking and representation that is done about nursing" (Cheek 1995a, p. 239).

In keeping with this, Gilbert (1995) asserts that:

> The nurse needs to be able to identify the discursive practices through which they as nurses are formed. For it is these, and their associated norms and values, which nurses then carry with them into their everyday roles. (p. 870)

Once such discursive practices are exposed, it may be possible to interrogate them, to explore which practices seem to dominate understandings of nurses and nursing, and which are relegated to the margins. Brown and Seddon (1996) note that the dominance of medicine over nursing lies in the fact that "society values the knowledge of processes of the body far more than the ability to care for the diseased body; hence not only is medicine given more authority, it is also more highly valued than is nursing" (p. 31). Research questions that arise from such analysis include how such a discursive position is maintained, who has an interest in such a maintenance and what the effect is of such discursive practices on how nurses are positioned in the health care sector.

Thus, postmodern-based research approaches offer the possibility for nurses to explore aspects of nursing care which otherwise might be taken for granted. In so doing, nurses may resist and even transform the effects of such discursive frames on understandings of nurses and nursing practice. New discourses about nursing may emerge which enable nurses to construct new subjectivities for, as Rabinow (1984) puts it, "maybe the target nowadays is not to discover what we are, but to refuse what we are" (p. 22). If the potential constraining effect of a particular discursive frame's dominance in the health arena is recognized, then it is possible for space to be opened up for other discourses or ways of thinking. This can add a multi-layered, multi-dimensional perspective to the aspect of health care reality in question. It is not a case of attempting to replace one discourse with another or of using one discourse to exclude others. Rosenau (1994) asserts:

> For post-modernists to assume, as did modern sociology, that there is one singular methodology [or discourse] appropriate for all circumstances risks repeating the same old imperialist attitude and advancing inappropriate claims to universality. Each side transforms their perspective into a totality. (p. 96)

The Clinic

Foucault was particularly interested in the relatively recent emergence of the clinic as central to health care practice. The birth of the clinic was possible because of a disease-based model of health care. Foucault (1975) asserted that the clinic was the institutionalization of the medical gaze: "a hearing gaze and a speaking gaze: clinical experience represents a moment of balance between speech and spectacle" (p. 115). By *gaze*, Foucault is referring to the act of seeing, or the way in which disease, illness and health care are thought about and viewed. The act of examining the body is a central tenet of the construction of health care around the locus of the clinic. In the examination, the body is made the object of the health professional's gaze. The body is scrutinized within the parameters of the scientific/medical discursive frame. The objectified body is then subjected to the regimes of truth and to the technologies of power created by the understandings of this discursive frame in the form of tests, procedures and further examinations. Examination of the body in this way allows for the development of further scientific/medical knowledge. The body is thus productive of certain forms of knowledge and in turn, subjugated to the discipline of these knowledges (Foucault 1977). Foucault (1975) suggests that the resultant disciplined body becomes a docile body which is the subject and object of the clinical gaze and its underlying premise of the legitimacy and authority of scientific/medical discourse.

In Foucault's analysis, the emergence of the clinic itself was only possible because of the emergence of certain types of discursive frames and associated knowledges. The clinic, in turn, operated to further produce certain types of knowledge whilst excluding others. Hence Long (1992) describes the clinic as:

> a mode of perception and enunciation that enables statements about disease. The clinic is a discourse because it is a set of rules and procedures within the field of inquiry....the clinic is more than a place where medicine is practiced, it is also a discursive practice, a language of health and disease. (pp. 119-120)

Foucault was particularly interested in the operation of power at various levels of society, including the level of the health care clinic. He conceived power as being capillary: operating in all levels and directions of society in an extensive network of power relations. This rejects the notion of power as emanating from the top. It also brings into question the notion that society can be divided into simplistic dichotomies, such as the dichotomy of those who have power and those who do not. As Foucault (1980) himself puts it:

> one should not assume a massive and primal condition of domination, a binary structure with "dominators" on one side and "dominated" on the other, but rather a multiform production of relations of domination. (p. 142)

Foucault is concerned with the effects of power at the very ends of the capillary network, that is, at the sites of its actions such as the clinic "rather than at some conjectured sovereign point (the state, the law, or wherever)" (Fox 1993b, p. 31).

Governmentality

This close relationship between power and knowledge can be seen in the connections between modern forms of governance and the discourses of human sciences such as medicine, psychiatry and law. Such government "implies all those tactics, strategies, techniques, programmes, dreams and aspirations of those authorities that shape beliefs and the conduct of the population" (Nettleton 1991, p. 99). According to Foucault (1979), governmentality is characterized by pervasive matrices of power which entail the surveillance and disciplining of both individuals and entire populations: the population is both subject and object of government. There is a network of power in that "the State is superstructural in relation to a whole series of power networks that invest in the body, sexuality, the family, kinship, knowledge, technology and so forth" (Foucault 1980, p. 122). Governmentality reinforces the "community" whilst at the same time (somewhat paradoxically), increasing individualization. Fox (1993b) defines governmentality as the "subtle, comprehensive management of life drawing both from a top-down exercise of power over conduct...with a subjectivity constituted in a sense of personal responsibility, rights, freedoms and dependencies" (pp. 32-33).

In such a conception, power is diffuse, anonymous and subtle, with its associated disciplinary regimes and techniques producing individuality. The individual is the site of the operation of powerful discourses, and is in effect a product of the inscription of such discourses. Thus:

> the individual is both the site for a range of possible forms of subjectivity and, at any particular moment of thought or speech, a subject, subjected to the regime of meaning of a particular discourse and enabled to act accordingly. (Weedon 1987, p. 34)

At the same time, registers of births and deaths and reports of certain diseases and other health-related statistics enable the monitoring of trends in disease and illness in entire populations. These trends can then be used to establish the norm and to further regulate and discipline the behavior of both individuals and entire populations, subjecting them increasingly to the gaze of the health professional's authority. According to Foucault (1982), "to govern, in this sense, is to structure the possible field of action of others" (p. 221). By its very nature, the exercise of this power relies on the knowledge of experts, for it is they who decide what is normal and abnormal within populations, and it is they who identify abnormality in individuals.

"Authorities of various sorts have sought to shape, normalize and instrumentalize the conduct, thought, decisions and aspirations of others in order to achieve the objectives they consider desirable" (Miller & Rose 1990, p. 8). The human body is thus a political body as well as corporeal, and it is "this political body which is the locus for the politics of health-talk, not the anatomical body which medicine and its adjunct disciplines have fabricated" (Fox 1993b, p. 24).

Foucault's analysis highlights the ongoing quest to normalize understandings and functions of the human body. There are "normal" functions of the body able to be delineated within normal understandings of appropriate ranges and limits. There are "normal" ways of practicing health care and treating illness/disease. Individuals are exhorted to attain, for example, "normal" ranges of height, weight and behavior. Disciplinary regimes are instituted for those who do not measure up according to the health gaze. Such disciplinary regimes involve individuals being under the constant scrutiny or gaze of a health "expert," the individuals themselves, or both the expert and individuals. Accompanying such scrutiny are disciplinary regimes such as diet, exercise or other more technical procedures all designed to restore the individual to the norm. The bodies of individuals are thus made visible and inscribed by the discourse of health professionals (Fox 1993b).

The capacity of experts in the human sciences to perform their functions of surveillance, categorization and intervention presupposes a set of power relations which enables them to carry out such activities. More profoundly, their discourses—the fields of possibility of their knowledge—about what counts as sickness or health, madness or sanity, criminality or lawfulness are the results of power relations. Medicine, with its knowledge of human bodies and its capacity to survey them, is an important mechanism of the modern disciplinary regime. The power of scientific/medical frames in contemporary health care is evident in that:

> Not only can these experts define the objects of their study, such as for example what constitutes a sick or insane client, but they also determine the limit of possibilities for the study, treatment and management of the objectified client. The power and control exercised by "experts" over clients-as-objects thereby constrain the types of discourse that are able to be developed about the client's condition. (Cheek & Rudge 1993, p. 276)

Using Foucauldian Concepts in a Study of Dental Health Care Practices: The Work of Sarah Nettleton

Using the research methods of archive analysis and interviews, Nettleton (1991) explored the concept of governmentality and its effect, focusing on dental hygiene and examination of children's teeth. She argues that "the discourse and practices that surround the mouth and teeth serve as an example of the mechanisms through which rule is exercised in Western society" (p. 98). Nettleton is particularly interested in exploring how the advent of the dental examination led to an aggregation of data on the "mouths of the population" (p. 101). From such statistics, knowledge was developed about population-based trends, and needs for dental hygiene and care.

This resulted in claims by dentists to expert knowledge and "wisdom" about the management and surveillance of dental health care, in order to evaluate, correct, rectify and restore to the norms derived from a comparison of the individual with the data about the "mouths of the population." Nettleton argues that concomitant with the development of such "wisdom" we see the rise of other agents, such as hygienists, health visitors and parents to assist in restoring the norm. Consequently, webs of governmentality are developed along with a vocabulary of "experts" situated at various sites such as the school, the dental surgery and the home. The development of such expert discourse is productive in that it enables knowledge claims and subsequent actions, yet also constraining in that it excludes other possible ways of viewing the issue.

Nettleton, following Foucault, explores how the home becomes both subject and object of scrutiny pertaining to dental hygiene and habits:

> There is no need for arms, physical violence, material constraints. Just a gaze.
> An inspecting gaze .... each individual thus exercising this surveillance over,
> and against, himself [sic]. A superb formula: power exercised continuously
> and for what turns out to be a minimal cost. (Foucault 1980, p. 155)

In light of such a gaze, and be scrutinized; the "ignorant" mother who is created as the result of expert discourses, and is able to be educated and to be subject and object of these expert discourses; and the "responsible" mother who complies with the expert discourse.

An important point made by Nettleton is that discursive frames used for the development of webs of governmentality are dynamic: they constantly change. "Wisdom, diligence and dentistry thus serve to individuals and whole populations are subjected to routines of dental hygiene. Nettleton outlines how certain moral discourses about the mother emerge from historical records of early education programs promoting sound dental routines. There are those of the "natural" mother who is the "natural" agent to effect change, scrutinize conceptualize and reconceptualize their object of government. Today their object is the thinking, active and productive patient and mother" (Nettleton 1991, p. 108).

Nettleton's analysis highlights how Foucauldian and postmodern analyses can illuminate and challenge aspects of the everyday reality of health care, many of which have become so taken for granted that they are assumed to be "normal" or the way things "should be." Her analysis also challenges the notion of an ever-progressive history—a challenge which, as we have seen, is at the heart of postmodern thought.

The Panoptic Gaze as Central to Contemporary Health Care

Foucault uses the metaphor of the panopticon to encapsulate his argument about the surveillance of individuals and even of whole populations by the gaze of "experts." The panopticon, as described by Jeremy Bentham, was a circular prison in which all cells were open and faced inwards towards a single central guard tower. All prisoners were thus under the potential scrutiny not only of the guard in the tower but of each other at any particular moment. Similarly, the guard could be scrutinized at any time by the prison governor. Consequently, a network of surveillance was created in which each individual was under the potential examination and gaze of a number of individuals at any one time. Not knowing when one was actually under scrutiny, or by whom, resulted in self-disciplinary, compliant and docile behavior because individuals acted as though they were under scrutiny at all times.

Foucault posited that such panoptic tendencies were evident in contemporary health care: in the examination of individuals by health professionals, in the individuals' self-policing of their own health, in the control of whole populations in the name of public health, and in the quest to normalize such populations. Individuals and populations could also be scrutinized by others and by themselves in regard to risk behaviors, lifestyle and susceptibility to certain diseases and illnesses. They stand perpetually before the gaze of a panoptical health connoisseur (Bartky 1988), who is able to scrutinize all aspects of their body and health. Foucault suggests that a consequence of such scrutiny is the development of docile bodies complicit in their own scrutiny and policing.

According to Foucauldian analysis, the examination of individuals by the gaze of experts such as those in the health care field is a disciplinary technique of power that invents "a new kind of individuality" (Hoskin 1990, p. 33), namely "the individuality...of the calculable [sic] man" (Foucault 1977, p. 193). Health practice is premised on confining or restoring individuals to the norm—a calculated and calculable norm beyond which anything or anyone is "other." In Foucauldian analysis, modern scientific/medical discourse is only one of many discursive frames within which health and illness might be conceptualized. The dominance of this discourse lies not in its rationality or logic but in the power that both underpins and maintains its discourse. It lies in the ability of its proponents to exclude others from practising different forms of health care and in its ability to relegate other ways of thinking about health care to just that—"other."

This is why Foucault (1984) states that:

> discourse is not simply that which translates struggles or systems of domination, but is the thing for which and by which there is struggle, discourse is the power which is to be seized. (p. 110)

Foucault: Some Concluding Remarks

It is important to note that Foucault resisted giving "a" method for doing Foucauldian-oriented research:

> Despite a concern with discourses as rule-governed systems for the production of thought, Foucault never sought to apply a particular system or to allow his own heuristics to congeal into a fixed, formal method. (Dean 1994, p. 14)

This possibly was to avoid giving the impression that there is "a" method for doing Foucauldian discourse-related research. To give "a" method would be to create another dominant discourse that could then be used to exclude other approaches.

Foucault's work has not been without its critics. Collins (1990) scathingly referred to Foucault as a theoretical "amateur" (p. 462) in that his theory was not developed or presented within conventional theoretical frames. However, as Agger (1992) points out:

> Collins does not recognize that Foucault would have loved to be called an amateur. Foucault implies that the professional/amateur distinction is a peculiar product of the discourse/practice of late capitalism, wherein unofficial knowledges are disqualified as unrigorous, undisciplined, unprofessional. (p. 126)

Further, Foucauldian analyses are often criticized as being nihilistic— pulling everything down and leaving little in their wake. As Waltzer (1988) puts it, "angrily he rattles the bars of the iron cage. But he has no plans or projects for turning the cage into something more like a human home" (p. 209). In relation to the health care context, Porter (Cheek & Porter 1997) echoes Waltzer's critique when he writes "while Foucauldian analysis can tell us a lot about what is wrong with where we are, it can tell us very little about where we should go" (p. 113). However, it could be argued that Foucault's major contribution is to expose the bars of what previously may have been a largely invisible, and thus taken-for-granted, iron cage. As Hoy (1991b) points out (drawing on the same analogy of the prisoner used by Waltzer):

> Foucault's voice may sound like that of the prisoner who wants out and cannot get out, but since Foucault is talking about our inability to get out of our own place in history, he is surely correct in this regard. (pp. 143-44)

Foucault never claimed to offer a total picture with all the answers. As Hoy (1991a) points out, Foucault rejected the "traditional philosophical goal of constructing a total theory that can explain the entire social reality" (p .5). Foucault does not offer the possibility of a power-less situation either in the health context or elsewhere. As Smart (1991) asserts:

It is clear therefore that in Foucault's terms there can be no power-free or power-less society, no millennial end of history towards which oppressed, exploited or dominated subjects may be led or guided, for relations of power, that is, ways of acting upon the actions of (other) acting subjects, are endemic in society. (p.169-70)

What Foucault does offer us, however, is a way of *understanding* power and its effects, rather than a grand vision of how power might be overcome. Instead of working to overcome or eliminate power entirely, it may be possible to work with it at different sites of the capillary relations of power that pervade any context, including the health care setting. In this way, Foucault may well offer optimistic analyses for resistance at the very edges of power networks—in the hospital ward or in the home, for example.

We are beginning to move into some complex arguments here that are beyond the scope of a text about postmodern and poststructural approaches in nursing and health care research. However, this brief and limited discussion has pointed to the complexity of Foucault's work. A fuller discussion of the possibilities and problems posed by the use of Foucauldian theory in nursing and health care is provided in an article "Reviewing Foucault: Possibilities and problems for nursing and health care" which I co-authored with Sam Porter. (Cheek & Porter 1997).

In this paper, which is written in the form of a dialogue between Porter and me on the relative merit of the contribution of Foucauldian theory to nursing and health care, many of the points briefly alluded to previously in this chapter are developed more fully. Details of the article are in the "Further Readings" at the end of this chapter. If you are interested in reading more on Foucault this article makes an ideal starting point. We concluded the article by cautioning against "bad short answers" (Hacking 1991, p. 27) to complex theoretical questions. Likewise, I wish to conclude this introduction to Foucault's work by reiterating that the discussion has necessarily been a brief overview. However, as is the case with our dialogue about the potential and problems of Foucault's work, "while the analysis offered here has indeed been modest in scope, the implications of what has been proposed are anything but" (Cheek & Porter 1997, p. 117).

USING A POSTMODERN THEORETICAL FRAME IN RESEARCH ABOUT HEALTH AND HEALTH CARE

This is all very well. Yet how can a theoretical frame such as postmodernism be used in research? What might a postmodern approach to research about a particular focus or area in health care look like? The best way to explore these questions is to look at ways in which researchers have drawn on postmodern approaches to inform their investigation of a particular health care issue. We have already explored how Nettleton used the concept of governmentality to explore aspects of dental care. The discussion to follow provides additional examples of the use of postmodern perspectives in exploring contemporary health care. In particular, it examines what a postmodern research lens can reveal about organizational strategies in contemporary health care, and the way in which such organizational strategies promote, and in turn are promoted by, certain understandings of health.

Fox (1993a; 1994), using ethnographic techniques and interviews, explored both the surgical operation and the surgical ward-round (i.e. in the United States "grand rounds") as organizational strategies that are constituted by the discourses of the various professionals who work within those strategies. He was interested in analyzing the way in which the organizational strategy itself (ie, the surgical operation or the ward-round) discursively constituted understandings of the role of the various health professionals. Thus, there was a dynamic interface between the discourses constituting understandings both of the organization of particular health contexts and of the practitioners working within those contexts.

In his analysis of the surgical operation, Fox (1994) focused on surgeons and anesthetists. These two groups of health professionals share many understandings of health care since both draw on the knowledge offered by the biomedical/scientific frame. Yet within the biomedical/scientific discursive field, as in any discursive field, there are many, often competing discourses. "Some will account for and justify the appropriateness of the status quo. Others will give rise to challenge to existing...organization and the selective interests which it represents" (Weedon 1987, p. 35). Which discourse is used at any point in time to frame and legitimate actions and exclude others is of interest. Thus Fox (1994) alludes to how the "surgeon and anaesthetist actively engage in fabricating their own versions of the reality of the patient in order to achieve their differing objectives" (p. 2). Fox's analysis points out that the discourses of these two groups of health professionals constitute the patient in very different ways in the operating theater. The anesthetist draws on a discourse of fitness with respect to the patient whilst the surgeon's actions are framed by a surgical discourse of disease and illness. Thus:

> An operation represents for the surgeon, the *desirable reduction in Illness* of a patient. For the anaesthetist it represents the *undesirable reduction in Fitness* of the patient. In any surgical procedure there will be a trade-off between reduction in Illness and reduction in Fitness. (Fox 1994, p. 10)

At times these discursive frames can lead to conflict between these two groups of professionals in terms of the meaning, desirable organization and outcome of an operation. Thus, if the anesthetist believes that the patient's fitness is being compromised by the surgical procedure he or she can use the discourse of fitness to challenge the surgeon's actions. Similarly, the surgeon can use the discourse of the desirable reduction of illness to override competing discourses about loss or reduction of the patient's fitness. Here we have an example of power as a capillary network—neither the surgeon or the anesthetist exercise a top-down approach to the power relations between them; rather, a network of power relations is in operation.

Fox (1993a) was interested in exploring the surgical ward-round as "an *organisational strategy* entered into by surgeons to achieve discursive hegemony" (p. 17). He did not analyse the ward round in terms of how, when and by whom it was conducted: rather, as with all discursive analysis, he looked critically at the practice of the ward-round *itself.* Questions which arise from such analysis include: what enabled an organizational strategy such as a ward-round to be established in the first place, and who or what subsequently enabled it to be maintained in that form? What part did the discursively framed understandings of the various health professionals involved in the ward-round, particularly the surgeons themselves, play in constructing the round? Conversely, how did the ward-round itself, and the discursive assumptions embedded within it, in turn frame understandings about the various health professionals? Finally, what about the patient? How does the way the ward-round is constituted position, and shape understandings about, the patient in relation to the other health professionals?

Fox (1993a) concluded that the ward round is an organizational strategy, structured around surgeon's understandings of disease, illness and healing which in turn operates to confirm those understandings. "I examine the ways surgeons manipulate ward-round interactions with their patients to their own advantage— to constitute and sustain their (surgeons') perspective on surgical healing" (Fox 1993a, p. 17). The ward-round organizes the interactions between surgeons and patients, defining what may or may not be said or done by surgeons, other health professionals and patients. As the ward-round is shaped by the discursive frames of the surgeons it "enables surgeons to set the agenda for their interactions with patients" (Fox 1993a, p. 22). Further, it can be used to construct "difficult" patients: that is, patients who do not fit the "normal" mode of behavior or "normal" role defined for them within the organizational strategies of the ward round.

Similarly, May, Dowrick and Richardson (1996) have explored the consultation between doctors and patients in general practice as an organizational strategy that frames the relationship between doctor and patient. May et al. focus on the ways in which the professional rhetoric of general practice has come to be organized around a very specific view of the possibilities that arise from this relationship.

The consultation, like the ward-round, is shaped discursively and in turn shapes the way the general practitioner and the patient are viewed by each other, by themselves and by others. The consultation and all that it entails in terms of setting, professional discourse and so forth is not the only way in which the interaction between patients and general practitioners might be organized. Yet, like the ward-round, it has become a taken-for-granted aspect of the organization of health care. Postmodern research approaches give the opportunity to ask such questions as why such organizational strategies exist, why they are maintained, and how they affect understandings of health and health care.

Here we are reminded of Foucault's exploration of the emergence of the concept of the clinic as the penultimate, discursively constructed organizational strategy underpinning contemporary health and health care understandings and practices.

This is not to suggest that there is no place for scientific/medical based discourse in health care. Such a suggestion would be absurd given that so many lives have been enhanced and saved by scientific and medical principles. However, it does suggest that the scientific/medical frame, as important as it may be, is not the *only* way of viewing or understanding contemporary health care. There are other possible discursive frames in which to view aspects of contemporary health care. As we have discussed earlier, nursing is one of these.

Focusing on nursing's relationships to medicine, Wicks (1995) explored the effects of the "truth" produced by dominant discourses shaping the organization and practice in a hospital ward and also looked at nurses' resistances to this "truth." Like Fox, she used ethnography as her research methodology, employing participative and non-participative observation and in-depth, semi-structured interviews. Also like Fox, she identified a hierarchy of discourses within the medical frame arguing that in more marginalized medical discourses, such as those of rheumatic disorders or palliative care, nurses are on a more equal footing. In dominant medical discourses such as surgery, nurses are seen "primarily as sources of information and the means by which medical orders are carried out" (Wicks 1995, p. 136). In keeping with the notion of a network of power, rather than a dichotomy between those who have power and those who do not, Wicks also documents and analyses some of the resistances of nurses to the "truth" of certain dominant discourses.

Thus, postmodern analysis offers the possibility for new and/or different discourses to surface in the health area. It enables the potential for the multi-dimensional and multi-perspective nature of health care to be represented through the frames of multiple discourses. A postmodern perspective allows for the analysis of why health care practices have been shaped in the way they are, and why certain players and practices in health care have been relegated to the margins, often designated as "other" rather than "another." This type of analysis may well form the basis of a postmodern-oriented research endeavor.

SUMMARY

This chapter has introduced the reader to the concept of postmodern thought as a critique of the assumptions that underpin modernist thinking. As such, postmodernist thought has been shown to problematize totalising descriptions and explanations of history, social structures and the health care context. Postmodern perspectives also problematize the researcher's position and his or her interests from the very conceptualization of the research to the methods of analysis employed when operationalizing the research.

Foucault's work provides a useful way of exploring what postmodern approaches can tell us about aspects of contemporary health care and health care practice. His concept of discourse—that is, certain ways of thinking and talking about reality—demonstrates the inextricable link between power and knowledge. Analysis of the impact of such discursive understandings opens up entirely new fields for research in nursing and health care which explore aspects of contemporary health care that have become taken for granted. The clinic and the examination are two such aspects.

The importance of the gaze in contemporary health care was explored using Nettleton's study of governmentality in dental care, which demonstrated the network of power surrounding the development of dental hygiene techniques and procedures. Of particular interest is the dynamic between the exercise of power at the macro level (such as in public health screening, establishing population norms for dental care and so forth) and the individual's complicity with such a gaze by adopting regimes of self-surveillance. Foucault's concept of panopticism extended the concept of the gaze, demonstrating the centrality of the medical examination as an outworking of the gaze in contemporary health care, and the production of docile individuals as objects of, and as subject to, such a gaze.

In the latter part of the chapter, examples of research that use these concepts were discussed in order to demonstrate how postmodern research can be operationalized in the world of practice and thereby provide understandings of that practice world. Fox's (1993a 1994) and May et al's (1996) exploration of certain organizational strategies in health care as discursively constituted provide a framework for our discussion. The discussion also explored the possibilities for other ways of viewing the organizational context of practice by postmodern analyses, including a nursing discursive frame.

The next chapter considers poststructural thought and its role in informing research in nursing and health care.

FURTHER READINGS

Best, S. & Kellner, D. (1991). *Postmodern theory: Critical interrogations.* New York: Guilford Press.

> Best and Kellner provide an introduction to postmodern thought and to a number of postmodern theorists. Of particular interest is Chapter 1, 'In search of the postmodern' which discusses both postmodern and poststructuralist perspectives, and Chapter 2, 'Foucault and the critique of modernity' which discusses some of Foucault's central ideas and the way in which these ideas contrast with modernist thought.

Cheek, J. (1997d). Postmodern theory and nursing: Simply talking trivialities in high-sounding language. In H. Keleher & F. McInerney (eds.), *Nursing matters.* (pp.79-95). Melbourne, Australia. Churchill Livingstone:

> This chapter provides a discussion of postmodern perspectives, through a contrast with modernist perspectives. It also explores some of Foucault's key concepts including those of power/knowledge, the notion of discourse (in particular, medical/scientific discourse), the clinic and the panopticon. These concepts are discussed in relation to the health care arena.

Cheek, J. & Gibson, T. (1996). The discursive construction of the role of the nurse in medication administration: An exploration of the literature. *Nursing Inquiry, 3*, 83-90.

> This article is a literature review of the nurse's role in medication administration. The authors argue that the practice of medication administration is discursively constructed. This is evident from an analysis of the procedures that nurses develop and institute as rules to guide nursing practice. The authors argue these procedures reduce nursing work to a series of rituals.

Cheek, J. & Porter, S. (1997). Reviewing Foucault: Possibilities and problems for nursing and health care. *Nursing Inquiry, 4* 108-119.

> Written in the form of a dialogue between two authors, this article addresses Foucauldian theory and its usefulness to nursing and health care research. It expands on and answers some of the critiques of Foucault discussed in this chapter.

Fox, N. (1993b). *Postmodernism, sociology and health.* Toronto: University of Toronto Press.

> Chapter 1 of Fox's book provides a discussion on the application of postmodern thought to the sociology of health and includes a discussion of the way in which medical and scientific knowledge results in a particular way of viewing the body. Chapter 2 is also relevant in that it discusses Foucault's concepts of governmentality and discipline.

Rabinow, P. (1984). Introduction. In P. Rabinow (ed.). *The Foucault reader* (p .3-29). New York: Pantheon.

Rabinow's introduction provides a good overview of the way in which Foucault positions his work in relation to modern thought. Issues discussed include power/knowledge, governmentality and the discursive construction of subjectivity. The book as a whole consists of extracts from Foucault's writings organized into a number of substantive themes, thus providing a good starting point for those new to Foucault's work.

Chapter 3

Thinking and Researching Poststructurally

OUTLINE OF THIS CHAPTER

In this chapter poststructural thought and the ways in which it can be used to explore health and health care are examined. The first section provides a succinct overview of what poststructural theory is and how it differs in emphasis from postmodern theory. Several concepts are also introduced, including the concept of text which is central to poststructural analysis and the concept of health care as textually mediated—that is, health care as shaped by and as shaping texts representing aspects of health care practices.

Discourse analysis as an example of a research approach used within a poststructural frame is then discussed at length. The chapter explores what discourse analysis involves and discusses ways in which discourse analysis has been applied in actual studies of health and health care. This includes studies of representations of disease and illness in the media and an analysis of the case notes constructed about two patients in a rehabilitation setting. Some key features of research which uses discourse analysis are then discussed, again drawing on an actual research project to illustrate and ground the discussion.

Deconstruction is then explored as another approach used within a poststructural research frame. The discussion of deconstruction focuses on the concept of binary oppositions. The chapter concludes by positing that the research process itself is a text able to be deconstructed.

POSTSTRUCTURAL THOUGHT

Like the term *postmodern, poststructural* is a contested concept and theoretical perspective. As stated in Chapter 1 of this book, poststructural perspectives have much in common with postmodern perspectives, so much so that some writers have used the terms synonymously. However, poststructural and postmodern perspectives differ in their focus and emphasis.

Unlike postmodern analyses which tend to be wider in scope and which focus on aspects of culture, society and history, poststructural studies have tended to concentrate on analyses of literary and cultural *texts*, where *text* refers to a representation of any aspect of reality. Therefore, the working distinction between postmodern and poststructural theoretical perspectives which will be adopted here is that posited by Agger (1991): "For my purposes here, poststructuralism...is a theory of knowledge and language, whereas postmodernism...is a theory of society, culture, and history" (p. 112).

Derrida (1976) asserts that "nothing is ever outside a text since nothing is ever outside language, and hence incapable of being represented in a text" (p. 35). Texts can be pictures, poems, procedures, conversations, case notes, art work or articles. Texts represent "conventionalized practices...which are available to text producers and interpreters in particular social circumstances" (Fairclough 1992, p. 194). Agger (1991) refers to these conventionalized practices as "the assumptions that every text makes in presuming that it will be understood" (p. 112) and goes on to point out that "these assumptions are suppressed, and thus the reader's attention is diverted from them" (p. 112). Thus, the way a text represents an aspect of reality, that is, the conventionalized practices and assumptions that underpin the shaping of the text itself, is of as much interest as what the text actually describes. In a later part of this chapter, we shall explore how practices and procedures in the health care area can be explored as texts, using poststructural perspectives.

It is crucial to recognize that in keeping with the way poststructuralism values plurality, fragmentation and multivocality, the term *poststructural* itself is plural. "It does not have one fixed meaning but is generally applied to a range of theoretical positions" (Weedon 1987, p. 19). Nevertheless, all poststructural perspectives interrogate language, meaning, and subjectivity (Weedon 1987). Poststructural perspectives challenge the notion that language is a neutral, objective, value-free conveyer of aspects of reality. Rather, they expose and interrogate language itself as being both constituted by, and constitutive of, the social reality that it seeks to represent. This includes the language used in texts such as the one you are reading now. Using a poststructural perspective, writers and readers of texts can recognize their own involvement and investment in the text that is produced.

For example, Agger (1991) argues that the very way we organize so-called "scholarly" writing represents certain views about what constitutes scholarship and how that scholarship should be conveyed. Importantly, it also enables claims of authority, and on the basis of that authority, the ability to dismiss other view points. Thus:

> How we arrange our footnotes, title our paper, describe our problem, establish the legitimacy of our topic through literature reviews, and use the gestures of quantitative method in presenting our results—all contribute to the overall sense of the text. (Agger 1991, p. 115)

In fact, as many of us will have found as reviewers of manuscripts for journals or research grant applications, it is often these unwritten rules and assumptions that influence our determination of whether or not the grant application or manuscript is "acceptable". Manuscripts and grant applications follow clearly delineated structures, often taken for granted as "the" way to write manuscripts or grants. However, in so doing it is easy to overlook the way that such structures embody the world views of those with power, such as funding bodies and editors, about the "right" way to produce particular genres of work. "The methods of representation...are themselves embedded inside a standpoint of power and authority" (De Montigny 1995, p. 213). Poststructural perspectives challenge such methods, focusing on the way texts are "structured by assumptions within which any speaker must operate in order to be heard as meaningful" (Ball 1990, p. 3).

Similarly, there are "correct" or accepted ways of acting and thinking in the health care arena. The very way health care and health care practices are organized represents certain views about what constitutes health care and about how that health care should be practised. These views also enable claims of authority and allow the ability to dismiss other viewpoints on the basis of that authority. Which particular ways of thinking about and of representing health care are afforded legitimacy in the health practice domain, and how such legitimacy is conferred, are of particular interest to researchers using poststructural perspectives to explore the health care arena.

Questions that might be asked by a researcher drawing on poststructural analyses about any representation of any aspect of health care reality include whether this is the only way this aspect of health care practice can be represented; why this representation is the one accepted as "normal" or "given"; what are alternate ways of representing the same reality; and why these ways are absent and/or marginalized and suppressed. Such questioning "calls into question claims to the autonomy, objectivity and political neutrality of medicine and public health" (Lupton 1993, p. 298), as language is exposed as "an important site of political struggle" (Weedon 1987, p. 24).

Already it is apparent that poststructural approaches lend themselves to a distinct research focus. The actual representations of health care practices and procedures, whether they are written, spoken or acted, become the data and the focus of the analysis rather than, for example, how many times a certain procedure or practice is carried out, and how effectively and efficiently. This is to take a step back in the depth of the research to be undertaken. Rather than accepting the reality of the clinical or health setting as a given, that very reality itself is made the focus of the research.

DISCOURSE ANALYSIS:
ONE METHOD WITHIN A POSTSTRUCTURALIST APPROACH

In Chapter 2 we explored Foucault's concept of discourse and how discursive frames shape understandings of health and health care. Using a poststructuralist lens with a focus on representation in texts, analyses of discourses that are present in texts representing aspects of contemporary health care can reveal much about the way in which our present understandings of health and health care have come to be what they are.

We will now explore discourse analysis as one method used in research that uses a poststructural approach. The analysis of discourses, or discourse analysis, "is not, or should not be, a "method" to be wheeled on and applied to any and every topic" (Parker 1992, p. 122). Rather, it involves a number of approaches. It is an interdisciplinary concept drawing on linguistics, cognitive psychology, anthropology, sociology and cultural studies, and is used in a variety of ways. However, this is in no way suggests that discourse analysis is a "free-for-all" where anything goes and anything can masquerade as discourse analysis. As Van Dijk (1997) indicates, all approaches to discourse analysis involve rigorous methods and principles of "systematic and explicit analysis" (p. 1), although the methods and principles may differ according to the approach to discourse analysis that is adopted:

> An analysis of discourse is a scholarly analysis only when it is based on more or less explicit concepts, methods or theories. Merely making "common-sense" comments on a piece of text or talk will seldom suffice in such a case. Indeed, the whole point should be to provide insights into structure, strategies or other properties of discourse that could not readily be given by naive recipients. (Van Dijk 1997, p. 1)

What then are the key features of any analysis of discourse? Discourse analysis is underpinned by the "notion of language as a meaning constituting system which is both historically and socially situated" (Cheek & Rudge 1994b, p. 59). Texts, whether they are books, articles, newspaper reports, interviews, observations or drawings, are embedded within discursive frameworks. They are constructed by the understandings of particular discourses and in turn they construct understandings in keeping with those discursive frames. "Meanings, as they occur in...text[s] are the product of dominant discourses that permeate those texts. Not only do powerful discursive frameworks provide meaning for the text, they actually frame the text itself in the first place" (Cheek & Rudge 1994b, p 61).

In discourse analysis then, "text is not a dependent variable, or an illustration of another point, but an example of the data itself" (Lupton 1992, p 148). Discursive analyses of texts are thus not simply descriptions or analyses of content: rather, they are critical and reflexive, moving beyond the level of common-sense.

Furthermore, discourse analysis situates texts in their social, cultural, political and historical context. Questions that may be asked include "Why was this said, and not that?" "Why these words?" and "Where do the connotations of the words fit with different ways of talking about the world?" (Parker 1992, p. 4). Texts are thus interrogated to uncover the unspoken and unstated assumptions implicit within them which have shaped the very form of the text in the first place.

Using two examples, we shall now explore how discourse analysis can be applied in research about health and health care. The first example looks at research into media representations of aspects of health, illness and associated health care practices. It shows how these representations reflect certain understandings and in turn create certain understandings of contemporary health care. The second example explores the way in which nursing work becomes textually mediated. It focuses on the discourses evident in case notes written about two rehabilitation patients, and in particular it focuses on whose voices are heard and whose voices are silenced in this process.

Discourse of Analysis, Example 1:
Analyzing Media Representations Of Health And Illness

The way in which disease and illness are constructed or represented in texts is "indicative of wider knowledge, belief, and value systems. Discourses on medicine, health, illness and disease construct realities in ways that are often taken for granted and invisible" (Lupton 1994c, p. 73). Thus, understandings of health, illness and disease cannot be viewed independently from the social context in which they are situated, since "knowledge reflects social, historical, and political phenomena" (Collyer 1996, p. 1).

One group of texts that have been very influential in framing the parameters for discussion of contemporary health issues, and even to some extent determining what is a health issue in the first place, is the publication of articles in the mass media. An exploration of the way in which health and health care issues are represented in such media gives important insights into how the media influence and shape societal attitudes towards health, towards those with certain illnesses, and towards health care practices. News, as reported and represented in popular media such as newspapers and magazines, reflects, and in turn creates, a particular view of reality. It is a "particular version of events" (Lupton 1994a, p. 29).

Gabe, Gustafasson and Bury (1991) analyzed the content of newspaper coverage on the issue of women's tranquilizer dependence. Their analysis highlighted the importance of taking into account ways in which mass communication can distort and bias understandings about dependence, how it can reaffirm stereotypical understandings about women's passivity and how it can thereby conceal crucial differences between groups or individuals who are dependent on tranquilizers.

In another study, Chrisler and Levy (1990) found after analysis of media content on pre-menstrual syndrome (PMS) that the messages conveyed by the media confused biologically-based premenstrual changes with the actual syndrome. Thus PMS became so inclusive in focus that it would be difficult for women not to find at least part of their experience recorded. Further, Stallings (1990) has demonstrated that perception of health risk occurs in and through processes of media and public discursive constructions. "Hence risk is never constant. It is created and recreated in discussion of events that are seen to undermine a world taken for granted" (p. 82).

Lupton (1994c) analyzed the way in which print-based media represented breast cancer and associated health issues. Her study looked at "dominant discourses evident in the Australian print media's reporting of breast cancer during a period in which the introduction of national mass mammographic screening programs was debated and ratified" (p. 74). She identified two potentially contradictory discourses framing the reporting at various times: the discourse of medical technology offering "the answer to diseases such as breast cancer" (p. 82) and the discourse of the "responsibility upon individuals for maintaining good health by preventative measures" (p. 82).

Lupton argues that one effect of such discourses enabling, yet paradoxically constraining, what is said about breast cancer and by whom, is the creation of the woman "at risk" who is both subject and object of technologies of power such as mammographic mass screening. This is often of the woman's own volition, with such volition arising from understandings created by the discursive frames of the taking of responsibility for one's health and the ability of medical technology to provide the answer. In such a discursive frame, the woman who does not have regular screening is portrayed as irresponsible. There is a "need" created for women to submit to these procedures. As Yoxen (1985) states, the analysis of such discursive framing should include questions about "how social and medical needs originate, how medical procedures and technologies are constituted, and what counts as expertise" (p.138).

The same author (1994c) cogently demonstrates the subtextual messages in the reporting of breast cancer about "women's role in society, women's bodies, and the nature of femininity" (p. 86). Similarly Sacks (1996), in an analysis of how media represented women and AIDS, found that "AIDS discourses on women focus on normative notions of sexuality, notions which are often conveyed through stigmatizing discourses about deviant women" (p. 70). In the reporting about AIDS, prostitutes are often represented as "indiscriminate, polluting to men and categorically different from 'normal' women" (p. 59). Such a discursive frame premised on a particular normative stance on sexuality serves to reinforce the "truth" about what is and what is not normal in terms of sexuality and women. Sacks posits that such truths have a normalizing and regulatory function, thus contributing to the way in which certain groups of women continue to be marginalized and "blamed" for not having enough self-control and self-discipline. "Such analysis casts light on the cultural meanings which the producers of media texts assume are shared by their audiences" (Lupton 1995, p. 93).

Other substantive areas explored by Lupton include media representations of AIDS and condoms (1994b), and the construction by the media of an "epidemic" of legionnaire's disease (1995). A consistently emerging theme is that news media can influence, and even set, health agendas in terms of quantity of the coverage and the content of the coverage. Media reports are shaped by the taken-for-granted understandings of health and disease, that is, by the discursive frames that underpin much of what is written and spoken about contemporary health care. In turn, media reports shape contemporary, taken-for-granted understandings of what health and illness are.

Stone's (1991) analysis of the way in which infertility and concomitant reproductive technologies have been represented in popular media demonstrates the changing nature of that representation and of the media's role in both creating and reflecting changing understandings of reproduction. This includes the definition and understandings of infertility itself:

> Most significantly, as they reported about new refinements and extensions of the assisted reproduction techniques, the media simultaneously helped to create a national "need" for infertility diagnosis (by the individual woman and by the expert). (Stone 1991, p. 316)

Thus, we see the emergence of new forms of experts and a new type of gaze and technologies of power (cf. Chapter 2, section 2.3.5) with respect to women and infertility:

> The idea of a "need" for new technologies to satisfy the "demand" created by the "reproductively impaired" was forged through links in discourse generated from multiple, interdependent institutions and organizations. The need was concretized over forty years. (Stone 1991, p. 326)

Consequently, contemporary representations of infertility are dominated by the idea that fertility is "an entirely *physiological* problem" (Stone 1991, p. 316).. Male infertility is represented as "something temporary, alterable and able to be controlled by the individual male's willpower" (p. 317), whereas:

> women, in contrast, are depicted as not quite so fortunate in their ability to reverse the consequences of their bad habits, and thus they are encouraged to "protect" their fertility long before they might even discover a problem with conception. (p. 317)

This includes self-surveillance of lifestyle to decrease the risk of infertility, especially as a woman ages. Stone also highlights the emergence of a discourse of fertility management evident in the reporting, outlining such techniques as taking one's temperature to ascertain ovulation and plotting one's ovulation on charts. Such a discourse normalizes these and similar techniques and enables the colonization of individuals by practices that are discursively constituted.

Conspicuously absent (or under-represented) in media reports is discussion on the links between environmental toxins and risks of infertility.

We have seen in this discussion of analyses on media representations of aspects of health and illness that discourse analysis can add to our understandings of contemporary health practices and of the way they came to be as they are. We will now explore a study based in an actual health care setting that used discourse analysis to demonstrate that everyday, often taken-for-granted procedures such as documenting in case notes in the health care context are textually mediated and that they represent certain views of the reality of health care.

Discourse Analysis, Example 2:
Analyzing Case Note Discursively

The study that forms the basis of this discussion was carried out by me and a colleague, Trudy Rudge (Cheek & Rudge 1994b; 1994e). We analyzed the case notes that were developed about two patients in a rehabilitation setting. The case notes were examples of health texts that were organized by, and in turn helped to organize, the dominant discourses framing the practice setting in which they were developed. The analysis took as its focus the interaction between the text (the case notes) and the context in which the text existed. A basic premise of this study was that nursing and other aspects of health care are textually mediated and that discourse analysis can provide insights into how text "both constitutes and reproduces the social act of nursing" (Cheek & Rudge 1994b, p. 61). In such analysis "our concern is not whether these are either a poor or good record of the events, but rather the nature of the reality produced by these texts" (Cheek & Rudge 1994e, p. 43). Such a focus moves the research beyond the descriptive and locates it in the realm of the discursive. Put another way, the focus is not so much on what is recorded as it is on why it is recorded, and conversely, why other things are not recorded. How did, and do, case notes come to be developed in the form they are, and why and how is such a form maintained?

How was this research actually done? As previously stated, the case notes of two randomly selected patients in a rehabilitation setting were analyzed. A rehabilitation setting was chosen because length of stay in this type of setting tends to be longer than in other health care settings; thus, it could be expected that the documentation and case notes developed about each patient would be substantial. In fact, both patients' notes in the analysis covered stays of four months. Further, by its nature, the rehabilitation setting is multidisciplinary. Consequently the notes developed reflect input from a large number of health professionals, thereby providing insights into the ways each professional writes about his or her practice independently and how they relate to the other health care providers in the rehabilitation context. All relevant ethical clearances were gained before the research commenced, including the consent of the two patients. The patients were Mrs. W, a 79-year-old woman who had fractured her femur in a fall, and Mr. H, a 63-year-old man who had suffered a stroke while on holiday.

Our broad research goals were to look at how the case notes and the accompanying "case" (that is, the patient) were represented textually in the notes. Case notes are "a deliberately 'crafted' document" (Poirier & Brauner 1990, p. 30) and reflect the influence of often competing discursive frames such as managerial, legal and medical discourses. Further, we wanted to look at how the actual space in the case notes was used or not used, and how it was managed by the various groups of health care providers writing the notes. The questions of who wrote, when they wrote, what they wrote about, and how they wrote were of great interest to us as this analysis offered important insights into how the groups of care providers interacted with each other and the patients in the webs of documentation developed. As Poirier & Brauner (1990) point out, although medical records (or in this study case notes) are constructed by diverse voices, "their notes are entered into the chart in a prescribed way, producing an organized record with a familiar sequence of information and events" (p. 30).

The constraints of space in a book such as this do not allow for an in-depth discussion of each patient's case notes and their analysis. Given such constraints, what follows is an illustration of some of the key points to emerge from this research from which we could give a sense of what type of analysis might emerge from such a study. The study has been reported in its entirety elsewhere (Cheek & Rudge 1994b; 1994e).

We began by looking at five specific areas. These were:

- the format of each entry—whether it was typed, handwritten or computer-generated;
- the ways in which the individual writers identified themselves—whether the entries were signed or not, and whether titles or qualifications were given;
- the similarities and differences between the various groups of health professionals in terms of content—what they wrote about and, of even more interest at times, what they didn't write about;
- how each group of professionals used the space in the notes—whether they wrote profusely, succinctly, or not at all;
- the form of language used: for example, was it the language of objective facts, using notations and symbols drawn from the discursive frame of the scientific/medical?

Each set of case notes revealed a common sequence of events in the initial construction of the notes. There was a record of what we termed the "rite of admission" for each patient in his or her notes. Such a rite was clearly situated in the frame of medical/scientific discourse where the "truth" of the patient's condition was established by examination by experts. In so doing, these experts used the authority given to them by scientific/medical discourse to establish the truth about the patient's condition. As a result of this examination, the patient can be located within such discourse—hence Mrs. W was described as "a fall who fractured her femur".

Once the patients were located, they were then able to be considered object of, and subject to, the medical/scientific discourse that defined them in the first place. Admission was thus concluded by the issuing of an identity number to each patient by which they could be monitored and scrutinized, and by the attaching of a wrist band to convey and confirm the identity of each patient. Further, additional statistics were collected about each patient to contribute to public health statistics and to meet government requirements for information about admissions and funding. At this point, the patients made their first, if not only, appearance in the notes. A record of consent given by each patient for treatment was found in each of the case notes following documentation regarding admission. However, there was no information about what each patient had been told about their condition or about what they had based their consent on.

Analysis of the notes reflected the centrality of the examination in contemporary health care provision. Each professional conducted his or her own examination of each patient and each group of experts used the examination(s) to situate the patient within their own field of expertise. At times, it was as though each professional was almost oblivious to what other care providers were doing, and the voices of each professional group seemed to speak "past one another, barely acknowledging each other's existence" (Cheek & Rudge 1994e, p. 45). In this respect, the case notes were comparable to Bakhtin's (1981) description of a novel: "a diversity of social speech types...and a diversity of individual voices artistically organized" (p. 262). Poirier & Brauner (1990) also used literary metaphors to describe the construction of the case report in terms of the various contributions to the report:

> The case report might more appropriately, in fact, be read as an anthology of short stories, a collection of world views which are brought together to address the same topic but which reflect the unique views of their individual authors. (p. 38)

Thus, it is not surprising that at times it is not clear who the audience is for either the case notes in general, or specific parts of the notes.

It was apparent that the notes assumed a privileged position in the health care setting. They were available only to "insiders". Not even the patient was openly granted the right to see these notes: the ownership of the notes was clearly with the health professionals. Further, the mystique associated with the symbols, abbreviations, jargon and shorthand used by exponents of medical/scientific discourse within the notes confirmed the exclusion from the notes of all but those privy to such knowledge. The patient as person effectively disappeared, irrelevant to such discursively framed notes. The patient was present only as defined "in relation to the contours of medical knowledge and practice" (May 1992, p. 591). The patient was thus reported as object: the source of information to be gleaned from examination. Further, the patient was subject to conclusions drawn from examination.

Nowhere was this more evident than in the following entries from Mrs. W's notes:

Claims [italics added] can't see out of right eye .... *claims* [italics added] she also struck occipital region of head .... *claims* [italics added] this is because of deteriorating R eye ....Viewpoint—no definite cause for falls. (Cheek & Rudge 1994e, p. 47)

Mrs. W's intimate knowledge of her own sight and her experience of her falls were discounted. The detached objective conclusion, following some sort of examination, was that there was no definite cause for her falls. As we have pointed out, in this instance the patient was:

constituted by the perceptions of the various "experts" recounting their perceptions of reality. Furthermore, these case notes [were] taken as objective, factual records of the patient's progress, whereas in actuality they represent[ed] one version of a number of possible realities. (p. 48)

The patient, being effectively excluded from access to what was written in the notes, had no right of reply.

The subjects/patients must then comply with regimes of treatment for their own good in the quest to restore "normality" according to the norms established by medical/scientific discourse. Such compliance is part of the development of the docile patient: "good" or "bad" patient can be gauged by the extent of conformity with directives (just like the "good" or "bad" mother in Nettleton's analysis (see Chapter 2: Using Foucauldian principles in a study of dental health care practices) and the responsible or irresponsible woman with respect to participation in breast screening, (see Discourse Analysis: Example 1 earlier in this chapter). For example, the nursing notes about Mrs. W record that she "obeys most commands" (Cheek & Rudge 1994e, p. 48). However, one nursing entry was particularly telling about the disapproving gaze on those who do not comply:

Nurse passing her room heard scraping furniture and investigated the noises, *rescued* [italics added] the patient and *reprimanded* [italics added] her...the client was *reminded* [italics added] that... .(Cheek & Rudge 1994e, p. 48)

The tone of the notes reflected in the use of words such as "rescued", "reprimanded" and "reminded" was disapproving and authoritarian. Whilst the nurse may be quite right that an elderly woman with a fractured femur is at risk of falling if she over-extends herself, the way in which the incident was recorded reflects the subjection of the patient to the norm in terms of what is deemed appropriate or "normal" behavior. What is conspicuously absent from such a record is how Mrs. W felt about, or reacted to, the incident.

In terms of such "conspicuous absences" in the notes, an analysis of the nursing documentation proved enlightening. Nurses tended to report the day's events not as they themselves had experienced it but in terms of the discourse of others, predominantly the medical/scientific.

Often it was others who reported important information drawing on nurses' experiences. For example, the following entry was made by a speech therapist in Mr. H's notes: "Ward staff have described his wife's considerable emotional difficulties, and it is clear that a certain lack of rapport currently exists between them" (Cheek & Rudge 1994e, p. 49).

Why did the nurses, who had made the important observation in the first place, not record it? Why was it left to the speech therapist to record this, and not to the group of health care providers who have the most constant contact with the patient and his family?

Parker and Wiltshire's (1995) analysis of the type of knowledge exchanged by nurses at handover provides insights into why this might be so. They delineated three modes of nursing practice knowledge communicated at handover: the nursing scan "reconnoitre" involving "constant scanning of the terrain of responsibility" (p. 157), the nursing gaze "savoir" and the nursing look "connaissance". They describe the nursing gaze (savoir) as "secondary and medically derived" (p. 166), involving objective technalized and medicalized knowledge about a patient's body,in which the patient is designated as an object, "the site of control" (p. 161).

Parker and Wiltshire argue that it is the nursing gaze, or savoir, that is afforded most prestige by nurses themselves. The nursing look is more affective. "The nurse's looking is not the cool or scientific inspection of the nursing gaze but a process of empathic understanding or reasoning in which patient and nurse are melded for a moment into one" (Parker & Wiltshire 1995, p. 162). Such knowledge is often considered unprofessional, subjective and taken-for-granted. It was the nursing look that identified the difficulties within Mr. H's family. However, because the knowledge associated with the more subjective look is not generally valued highly by nurses themselves, nurses do not record these difficulties. Instead, their documentation often adopts the tone of the cool, judgmental inspection underpinning the nursing gaze. The following entry in Mrs. W's notes reflects the nursing gaze, as opposed to the more empathic look which was marginalized and absent from the notes:

> Up to commode x2 overnight. Happy to rely on assistance from staff. More than was seemly....She seems only to be severely lacking in motivation (Cheek & Rudge 1994e, p. 50).

The analysis of these two sets of case notes,with respect to the nursing voice and to voices within that nursing voice supports Parker and Wiltshire's (1995) contention that:

> because of the dominance of the medical voice in the hospital context, supported as it is by the disciplinary power of medical knowledge, it is not surprising that the nursing voice is somewhat muted. (p. 166)

However, possibly even more surprising is how discourse analysis of case notes reveals that nurses are actually complicit in such a muting or silencing of aspects of the nursing voice! As Cheek & Rudge (1994b) assert:

> It is not just that the…[case notes]…*represent* nursing as a process that is technical in its intent, but that these practices are *constituted* by the taken-for-granted nature of the authority embedded in both the content *and* form of such texts. (p. 66)

From the study discussed it is possible to see the potential that discourse analysis has to offer analyses of specific procedures in health care and health care practices. I have illustrated the type of data and analysis that might form part of a discourse analysis of the documentation that is routinely developed about patients in health settings and which otherwise is unlikely to be analyzed but taken for granted as a neutral record of a patient's experience. In no way should the study be viewed as an argument against documentation. Rather, it should be viewed as a to strip away the veneer of:

> neutrality and objectivity articulated within documents such as case notes, in order to expose the dominant discourses shaping the communication in them ….by exposing the power of deeply engrained dominant discursive frameworks, we enable the possibility of resistance. (Cheek & Rudge 1994e, pp. 51-52)

Thus the study is an exploration of how case notes have been shaped predominantly by certain discourses and especially by the scientific/medical.

The examples that have been discussed throughout this chapter demonstrate how discourse analysis can be used to explore and expose health care practices as textually mediated, and in so doing can open up the way for other possibilities for those practices. As Poirier and Brauner (1990) so succinctly put it:

> The pen may not be mightier than the stethoscope in this instance; but the more fully aware health professionals are of the power and individuality of their words, the more conscious they may become of their own beliefs and influence—and the role of that influence in medical education and patient care. (p. 39)

"Doing" Discourse Analysis:
Key Features Of Research Using Discourse Analysis

We have discussed how discourse analysis has been used in a variety of studies about aspects of contemporary health care. We will now consider some key features of research that uses discourse analysis. Parker (1992) outlines four key features, or stages, of discourse analysis. However, as he does so he is careful to point out that there is no set "recipe" for discourse analysis.

Rather, research into discourse "should be led by the issues and problems that are to be addressed and, where possible, by research participants" (p. 122). Further, as we have seen, there are many types of texts. Discourse analysis applies to texts generated from, for example, interviews, group discussions and newspaper articles. With these points in mind, the four stages/features of discourse analysis posited by Parker are as follows:

1. Introduction.

This is where the study is positioned with respect to its relationship to other works on the substantive area. These works are drawn from a "traditional" search of the literature, as they are in any other research undertaking, and do not include only studies using discourse analysis. Further, the type of texts to be analyzed as well as the types of questions/issues driving the research are discussed in order to contextualize the research.

2. Methodology.

In this section detail is given about the specific texts to be analyzed. Why these texts and not others were chosen as the focus of the study is an important consideration to be discussed here. Information is also given about how these texts will actually be obtained (e.g. by interview or collection of articles. As in any research plan, detail is needed about the type of interviews conducted or about the type of article collected.

3. Analyses.

Parker outlines the coding of the data (which, in discourse analysis, is the text itself) under different discourse headings. Of particular interest to the analysis is any absence of possible discursive frames. That is, what ways of speaking and thinking about the reality in question are not present and why might that be so?. There is no set way of doing such analysis and Parker, in keeping with Hollway (1989), suggests that it is inevitable that a degree of intuition must be employed.

4. Discussion.

In this section the analyses are linked to other material in the area in order to draw out points of discussion about the substantive area under scrutiny. This section also involves "reflection on the issues raised by the method including, crucially in the case of material in which you participated (such as interviews), the position of the researcher" (Parker 1992, p. 123).

Parker's book also has an interesting section in Chapter 6 that looks at a range of areas and ways in which discourse analysis has been employed, and you may find it useful to read this. However, a key suggestion made by Parker is that "perhaps the best way to get a feel for forms of discourse is to look at how analysts actually deal with texts" (p. 127). This is sound advice.

Discourse analysis can be talked about and described *ad infinitum*, but examining actual studies clearly demonstrates how discourse analysis may be used and its potential for informing understandings of health. With this in mind, we will explore another study that has used discourse analysis to explore an aspect of health care. The object of such an exploration is to demonstrate how Parker's four stages can form the framework for an actual research study. In so doing, the aim is to get a "feel" for discourse analysis.

A colleague (Terri Gibson) and I became interested in the way that nurses and the nursing role, in relation to the administration of medications, were represented in the health literature. Our interest arose from our involvement in a large funded study that sought to ascertain registered nurses' perceptions about their role in the administration of medications. In the study, we asked these nurses to relate practice situations or critical incidents they had experienced in relation to administering medications. Analysis of their responses led to the development of a framework from which to view the nurse's role in medication management. This framework then informed the development of a self-directed educational package designed to promote the quality administration of medications by nurses. The study has been reported in depth elsewhere (Beattie, Cheek & Gibson 1996; Cheek 1997c) and is not the focus of the discussion here.

The focus here is what we found when researching the literature to ascertain what had been written about nurses and their role in the quality use of medications. This led us to carrying out a discourse analysis of the published literature pertaining to nurses and medication administration at the same time as we were part of a team conducting the large funded project. It became, as it were, a study within a study! I will now explore what we did when analyzing the discourses present in the literature, using Parker's (1992) four stages as a loose framework. It is interesting to note that when we were doing the study of the literature we did not set out to use these four stages as such, but what we actually ended up doing was in keeping with them.

In the introductory phase of the study we looked at what had been written about the role of nurses in the administration of medications. We focused on the literature related to nurses and medications from the mid-1980s to the present. These articles were the texts to be analyzed in our study. Our questions and issues for the research were derived from our impression that the focus of most of these articles was on procedures to govern and regulate the behavior of nurses. Our methodology was straightforward. It involved searching the CINHAL (Cumulative Index of Nursing and Allied Health) and MEDLINE databases for articles pertaining to nurses and medication administration from 1985 to 1995, and then obtaining copies of the articles. These databases, and not others, were chosen as these were the two databases that were expected to list articles in the relevant area.

The effect of dominant discourses on the way nurses were represented in relation to medication administration was evident from a very early stage of the analysis. We (Cheek & Gibson 1996) noted that:

> The literature draws heavily on the discursive frameworks of the scientific and legal, with much writing devoted to the consequences of drug errors, but only as they apply to the bodily functioning of the client (scientific/medical discourse) or to the responsibility of the nurses (legalistic discourse) (p. 85),

and

> research [into medications] has generally been framed within the discourse of science and has focused on identifying error rates and categories of error, and their relationship to procedural and system deficiencies. (p. 85)

Thus, early on, two discourse headings emerged: scientific/medical and legal.

In keeping with discourse analysis, whilst accepting that knowledge about the error rate of medication administration by nurses is important, we asked ourselves what was missing or absent from these articles. We found that the voice of nurses themselves was largely absent. For example, there was no reporting of why nurses said errors occurred, or about whether nurses believed administration procedures were effective. On the other hand, the opinions and voices of managers, administrators, lawyers, doctors and even of pharmacists were prominent in discussions about nurses and the administration of medications.

Finally, in discussing our analyses, we linked our findings about the dominant discursive frames in terms of how nurses and the administration of medications are represented to wider issues such as the production of self-surveillance and docility in nurses:

> Nurses are under the constant scrutiny of patients who may well know their medication regimens better than the individual nurse in question. Further, nurses constantly scrutinize patients...additionally they [nurses] scrutinize each other in the guise of double checks, incident reports, medication variance reports, quality assurance audits...these rituals in effect serve to act as mechanisms by which nurses can and do police each other, and reinforce the notion of control and docility. (Cheek & Gibson 1996, pp. 86-87)

This led us to apply Foucault's (1977) concept of the panoptic gaze to the analyses.

We concluded our research by exploring the concept of the subject position of the nurse in terms of the discursive frameworks that are developed about nurses and the administration of medications. As discussed previously in this book, there are a number of possible subject positions that can be taken within any discursive frame. This is so with respect to the subject position of nurses within the scientific/medical and legal discursive frames that shape the role of the nurse in medication administration. Thus, by exposing the discourses operating to create understandings of nurses with respect to medication administration, our research enables possibilities for nurses to resist being positioned by these discursive frames, and to recognize that other subject positions are possible. The potential for the emergence of a nursing discourse is enabled. We concluded with a challenge to nurses "to identify such points of resistance and develop alternative discourses of medication administration" (Cheek & Gibson 1996, p. 88).

Discourse Analysis—Some Concluding Comments

Health and health care are textually mediated in terms of the understandings that both frame texts and are conveyed by those texts. We have seen how analysis of ways in which this is done raises important issues with respect to the reality of health care practice. Far from being removed from understandings of practice and therefore unable to contribute to them, discourse analysis challenges the everyday, often taken-for-granted realities of the health care setting from the role of the professionals in it to the documentation developed about patients.

However, like any research technique and approach, discourse analysis has limitations. As we have seen, discourse analysis draws on traditions from many disciplines, each of which has its own particular emphasis on the way discourse analysis is operationalized. Because it allows for multiple perspectives, such diversity can be a strength of discourse analysis: but it can also be a limitation if the approach used is poorly defined or not contextualized in terms of its theoretical origins. In addition it is important that discourse analysis does not remain only at the micro-level of analysis but be extrapolated to the macro level. It must consider the social and political realities of the context by which the text is mediated and which in turn it mediates. As Cheek & Rudge (1994b) point out:

> Although these links between the macro and micro perspectives are important in order that discourse analysis can provide rigorous forms of analysis, these links do not as yet present a coherent perspective. This, Van Dijk considers, is the project of discourse analysis in the 1990s. (p. 65)

Finally, it is important to point out that readers of texts are not passive consumers of those texts: rather, individuals are active readers of texts. As Ang and Hermes (1996) (after Hall 1982 and Gledhill 1988) declare, "'Reading' is itself an active, though not free, process of construction of meaning and pleasure, a 'negotiation' between texts and readers whose outcome cannot be dictated by the texts" (p. 113). Every textual reading (including this one) is a negotiated one (Kaplan 1992) in the sense that there is a negotiation on the part of the reader between the viewing position created by the text and the understandings that the reader brings to that text (Cheek 1996). Yet, as Frazer (1992) points out, "all too often theorists commit the fallacy of reading 'the' meaning of a text and inferring the ideological effect the text 'must' have on the readers (other than the theorists themselves, of course!)" (p. 186).

Thus, research into the readers of texts in the health care arena is needed to investigate the negotiated readings of those texts that are actually adopted. Discourse analysis of texts is somewhat speculative if the way texts are read is not investigated.

Nevertheless, discourse analysis remains a useful and important research approach that is able to expose the way in which health texts frame the reality of contemporary health care. It is thus a useful way to explore the paradox that exists with respect to these texts:

> The paradox is that not only can textual portrayals and analyses of health care practice enhance our understandings of health, they can also limit them if we do not recognise that the viewing position adopted, from which to frame our analysis, can have the effect of confining our understandings to certain parameters. (Cheek 1995b, p. 60).

DECONSTRUCTION: ANOTHER APPROACH TO RESEARCH FROM POSTSTRUCTURAL PERSPECTIVES

Deconstruction is another approach that is associated with the exploration and interrogation of texts using poststructural perspectives. Poststructural perspectives, and in particular deconstruction, are often associated with the work of the French theorist Jacques Derrida, even though he, like Foucault, is careful not to classify his work as belonging to any particular theoretical orientation. As Bloland (1995) puts it:

> The Derridian strategy is to search out and illuminate the internal contradictions in language and in doing so show how final meaning is forever withheld or postponed in the concepts we use. The means for carrying out this project is deconstruction. (p. 526)

However, it is important to recognize that Derrida has not elaborated "a single deconstructive method" (Agger 1991, p. 112). Rather, the term deconstruction represents a range of approaches each with its own emphases. Consequently, deconstruction does not represent a unitary concept; it involves a multiplicity of fields and styles:

> To present "deconstruction" as if it were a method, a system or a settled body of ideas would be to falsify its nature and lay oneself open to charges of reductive misunderstanding. (Norris 1991, p. 1)

Norris goes on to point out that at times, the term deconstruction tends to suffer from a fairly loose usage to refer to any critique of existing social structures.Nevertheless, despite ambiguity and plurality in the way the term "deconstruction" is used, all deconstructive approaches have the same purpose. Rather than seeking to find "the" meaning within, or of, any text, they seek to challenge the very meanings and the assumptions on which those meanings are founded:

> Methodologically, deconstructionism is directed to the interrogation of texts. It involves the attempt to take apart and expose the underlying meanings, biases, and preconceptions that structure the way a text conceptualizes its relation to what it describes. (Denzin 1994, p. 185)

Thus, deconstruction involves a certain way of thinking about texts and a certain way of "reading" them: not to find "the" meaning of that text but to trouble the assumptions underpinning the text. Deconstruction involves looking at the representation of reality in the text as a partial representation (Feldman 1995) exploring silences and gaps in the text and what they reveal. Thus, deconstruction is "less method than perspective, a kind of interpretative self-consciousness" (Agger 1992, p. 95).

Agger (1992) has highlighted some of the assumptions implicit within a deconstructive approach and it will be useful to briefly review his argument here. The first assumption is that culture is a text and can therefore be interrogated as a text: "the boundary between the textual world and the social world fades once we subject culture to a deconstructive reading" (Agger 1992, p. 98).

The second assumption is that deconstruction aims to locate the author. By this Agger is alluding to the unwritten and unspoken assumptions that the author has made by selecting what will, and conversely will not, be said or written in the text and by determining what form the text itself will take. Thus the text is stripped of claims of objectivity and the author's influence is exposed.

For example, in carrying out scientific research and writing scientific research reports, standard, supposedly objective, scientific conventions are followed in terms of the way that both the research and the subsequent research report is structured. Deconstructive approaches trouble this concept, arguing that in writing and reading science:

> the science writer buries the subjectivity of the writer underneath the heavy prose of methodology, allowing technical language and the figural gestures epitomizing science to take control of the text. The writer's deep assumptions about the nature of the world are suppressed underneath the technical surface of the text, hidden from the community of science and thus protected from external challenges. (Agger 1992, p. 102)

The third assumption identified by Agger in a deconstructive approach is that every cultural text is undecidable: the meaning is never given, but is open to challenge and contestation. Thus, another assumption is that a deconstructive approach seeks the aporias, that is the blind spots, omissions, tensions, circumlocutions and contradictions, in every text. Agger (1992) refers to these as the "internal fissures and fault lines" in a text (p. 102). A deconstructive reading pries open such fissures and fault lines to reveal the underlying subtextual frames of the text, some of which may actually be in competition with one another. Thus, another assumption of deconstructive approaches identified by Agger is that the subtext is turned into text.

A deconstructive approach reads at the margins and views "many overlapping and cross-cutting texts—texts within, and beyond, texts, stories within, and beneath stories" (p. 108).

Finally, a deconstructive approach assumes that reading "writes", "because there is no way to develop readings outside of language and textuality" (Agger 1992, p. 105). In so doing, deconstruction challenges the privileging of the written text over the reading of that text. Every act of reading any text creates a new and different text. Thus, the reading of any text and the criticism that accompanies it transforms that text, opening it to "new versions of itself by bringing to light its hidden assumptions and inconsistencies" (Agger 1992, p. 96).

The Concept of Binary Oppositions

The notion of privileging the written text over the reading of that text highlights one of the very specific points in Derrida's deconstructive approach. This is the concept of binary oppositions, whereby one term is always prior or dominant to the other which is secondary or subordinate. For example, in the assumption of the authority of written text as opposed to the authority of the reading of that written text there is a binary structure of meaning and value in operation. "Written" is the prior or dominant term, and "reading" the secondary or subordinate term. We can express this binary opposition as written-read. Other common binary structures in place are masculine-feminine; doctor-nurse; theory-practice; mind-body. In all of these structures the first named term is the dominant term which is afforded primacy over the:

> secondary "weaker" or derivative term in the pair that is defined in terms of "not the dominant" .... however, the definitional dynamic extends to the primary term as well in that it can only sustain its definition by reference to the secondary term. Thus the definition and status of the primary term is in fact maintained by the negation and opposition of the secondary partner. (Cheek, Shoebridge, Willis et al. 1996, p. 189)

The repression or deferral of the subordinate term is thus crucial for the governing position held by the superior term. Figure 3.1 gives an interesting and somewhat humorous analysis of the effect of reversing common binary pairings.

Derrida's thesis is that binary pairings are not "natural" or "normal": rather, they are constructions which reflect embedded assumptions about value and status. Thus, part of the deconstructive venture is to uncover such pairings and to expose their effects. In so doing, "binary oppositions thus become analytical sites of ongoing struggle and contestation" (Cheek & Rudge 1994c, p. 19).

It is by exposing and reversing common binary oppositions that the effect of such oppositions on our concept of social reality is revealed. Wajcman's (1994) clever parody of a medical research report into the testing of a new contraceptive powerfully demonstrates the effect of such oppositions on our concept of social reality and what reversing or displacing them can reveal.

The newest development in male contraception was unveiled recently at the American Women's Surgical Symposium held at Ann Arbor Medical Center. Dr Sophie Merkin, of the Merkin Clinic, announced the preliminary findings of a study conducted on 763 unsuspecting male students at a large midwest university. In her report, Dr Merkin reported that the new contraceptive—the IPD—was a breakthrough in male contraception. It will be marketed under the trade-name 'Umbrelly'.

The IPD (or intrapenile device) resembles a tiny folded umbrella which is inserted through the head of the penis and pushed into the scrotum with a plunger type instrument. Occasionally there is perforation into the scrotum but this is disregarded since it is now known that the male has few nerve endings in this area of his body. The underside of the umbrella contains a spermicidal jelly, hence the name 'Umbrelly'.

Dr Merkin declared the 'Umbrelly' to be statistically safe for the human male. She reported that of the 763 students tested with the device, only two died of scrotal infection, only twenty experienced swelling of the tissues. Three developed cancer of the testicles, and thirteen were too depressed to have an erection. She stated that common complaints ranged from cramping and bleeding to acute abdominal pain. She emphasised that these symptoms were merely indications that the man's body had not yet adjusted to the device. Hopefully the symptoms would disappear within a year. Dr Merkin and other distinguished members of the Women's College of Surgeons agreed that the benefits far outweighed the risk to any individual man.

Figure 3.1: Exploring the Effects of Reversing Binary Oppositions

SOURCE: Technological a/genders: Technology, culture and class, (p. 10), Wajcman, J., 1994. In L. Green and R. Guinery. (Eds.), *Framing technology: Society, choice, and change*. St Leonards, NSW: Allen and Unwin. Copyright 1994 by Allen & Unwin. Reprinted with permission.

To illustrate the possibilities afforded by this approach, try reversing the order of the terms in the binary pairings discussed previously. What would the effect be in the health practice setting of the following reversals: practice-theory; nurse-doctor; body-mind? Why aren't these the binary pairings which are taken for granted? How are the primacy of certain terms and the subordination of others maintained? Who has an interest in such a maintenance of binary pairings? Figure 3.2 extrapolates these ideas to the university setting to further illustrate the concepts we have been exploring.

Here is how the 'study culture' of a university builds meanings—and so behaviours—for the academic staff versus the students.

A Theory readings	B Student exercises
: concentrated theory in 'readings'	: the 'unlearned' student
: content presence	: content absence
: question posing	: question answering
: expert	: novice
: source for expertise	: source for raw data

Now try contesting this view!

A Student exercises	B Theory readings
: the experienced practitioner	: the second-order theorists
: content presence	: inherited content
: question creating	: question processing
: expert	: intellectual order
: source for knowledge	: source for data collation
: practical	: abstract

What has happened? Is this 'contested' reading of 'who is more important' as powerful as the one above it?

Figure 3.2 Binary oppositions in the study culture: the academic/the student

SOURCE: *Advanced Practice Studies 3: Nursing Practice as Textually Mediated Reality*, (p.24), J. Cheek & T. Rudge, 1994a, Underdale: University of South Australia. Copyright 1994 by the University of South Australia. Reprinted with permission.

These are important questions which can lead to many interesting and fruitful research undertakings. Such research challenges the very concepts and understandings that are at the core of health practice, yet they have often been taken for granted to the point that they are often assumed or are even invisible. Deconstructive approaches enable us to ask completely different sorts of questions in the research process. Often the focus and/or data of such research are what is assumed as the starting point in more "traditional" research undertakings.

As Spivak (1976) asserts, in doing this type of research the text, which can be any representation of aspects of reality including health care, "becomes open at both ends. The text has no stable identity, stable origin...each act of reading the 'text' is a preface to the next" (p.xii).

Deconstruction:
Exploring a Binary Opposition in Practice

We will now briefly explore a binary opposition which operates to create and sustain understandings of a concept that is central to nursing and health care practice: care itself. Thomas (1993), drawing on the work of Gillian Dalley (1988), comments on the dual meaning of care: caring for someone and caring about someone. Caring for and caring about are potentially oppositional terms. Caring for someone has tended to become enshrined in the professional discourses and the techniques of the so-called "caring" professionals. Here, care is often reduced to what must be done to people in order to care for them. Accompanying such professional discourses are expectations about the way in which carers will behave when caring for someone. To act in a professional manner often means to detach emotionally from patients, to keep a professional distance. Hence, to a large extent the definition of caring for someone becomes defined in terms of expunging much of what is bound up in caring about someone.

Building on the binary opposition of caring for/caring about, Fox (1995) has explored what he terms the "vigil" and the "gift" with respect to the outworking of care in the health professions. The vigil of care is linked to understandings embedded in the discourses surrounding caring for someone. Thus, Fox defines the vigil as:

> the continual subjection of care's clients and increasingly, all aspects of the environment in which they live to the vigilant scrutiny of carers, and the consequent fabrication and perpetuation of subjectivities as "carer" and "cared-for". (p. 112)

In many ways, Fox's concept of the vigil of care is close to the nursing gaze (savoir) identified by Parker and Wiltshire (1995) and discussed earlier in this chapter. The vigil of care not only constructs what the role of the carer should or should not be (usually with reference to aspects of caring about), it constructs the patient. "The vigil of care is the disciplinary technology which, through discourses of professionalism and theory, fabricates and inscribes those who are cared-for" (Fox 1995, p. 115). Within the vigil, as in the gaze, is the element of scrutiny and surveillance which enablesthe carer not only to care for the patient in the institutional setting but to extend such care to the home and to aspects of individuals' lives. We already saw this when we discussed Nettleton's analysis of the emergence of professional discourses of caring for dental health.

In contrast to the vigil of care, Fox identifies the gift of care, which draws on caring about rather than caring for. Here Fox draws on Cixous' (1986) work. Cixous has theorized two realms: the "gift" and the "proper". She identifies the properties of the "proper" as masculine and those of the "gift" as feminine. The "proper" is identified with "property, propriety, possession, identity and dominance" (Fox 1995, p. 116). Conversely, Fox lists some characteristics of the gift: "generosity, trust, confidence, love, benevolence, commitment, delight, patience, esteem, admiration and curiosity" (p. 116). He notes:

> how few of these words are part of the discourse of professional care, which indeed suggests relations which could be seen as *un-professional* and inappropriate to the highly theorised, formalised care documented in textbooks, in which the carer/cared-for distinction is so strong and so impenetrable. (p. 116-17)

We are reminded here of Parker and Wiltshire's identification of the nursing look (connaissance). The nursing look as opposed to the nursing gaze is premised on caring about, feeling empathy for, and being with the patient. Yet like the gift, the nursing look is not given primacy: it is relegated to the margins as not being part of the professional discourse of nursing and the care provided by nurses.

An exploration of the binary opposition of caring for and caring about enables us to explore many of the tensions and contradictions that face nurses and other health professionals in their everyday practice. By identifying the effect of primary terms such as caring for, we are able to reflect on what the effect might be of reversing the primary term with its subordinate term, in this case caring about. As Fox (1995) concludes:

> we can point to the kinds of activities within caring which constitute the vigil, and reflect that there is always the possibility of resistance, that things can be different, and take it from there. (p. 123)

Thus, an interesting question on which to reflect is what the effect would be of reversing the caring for/caring about binary opposition on notions of health care and health care practice.

Research as a Text That Can Be Deconstructed

At this point we will pause to consider aspects of research methods and research processes as texts which can be deconstructed and subsequently we will see what the effect of such a deconstruction might be. Are there binary oppositions in place in terms of the values and emphases inherent in assumed understandings of research? Think of the debate that has surrounded qualitative versus quantitative approaches. Is a binary pairing in operation—namely quantitative/qualitative—in which quantitative approaches have been afforded primacy by many research "authorities" and qualitative approaches have been defined largely in terms of what they are not? Think also of the central binary pairing that has so influenced both research and claims to research "validity": objectivity/subjectivity. The effect of such a dichotomy has been to privilege certain so-called neutral and value-free approaches to research.

However, as we have seen, claims to being neutral and value-free can hide assumptions about world-views and may operate to conceal other ways of viewing or researching the same reality.

Research methodologies themselves are texts which are framed by, and in turn frame, understandings about the nature of knowledge and about certain views of the way to research any given aspect of reality. This is not to deny the importance of research methods, including traditional scientific/empirical approaches. Rather, it is to explore the concepts and assumptions embedded in any methodology employed and to consider the effect that these assumptions have on the research undertaken, including the way it is reported. Such a deconstructive project opens up many possibilities:

> Methodology can be read as rhetoric, encoding certain assumptions and values about the social world. Deconstruction refuses to view methodology simply as a set of technical procedures with which to manipulate data. Rather, methodology can be opened up to readers intrigued by its deep assumptions and its empirical findings but otherwise daunted by its densely technical and figural nature. (Agger 1991, p. 114)

Thus, deconstructive approaches are effective for "interrogating taken-for-granted assumptions about the ways in which people write and read science" (Agger 1991, p. 106). Such interrogation is crucial if other approaches are to be enabled to surface. As Agger points out, many published research reports:

> rely on the rituals of methodology in order to legitimate a certain form of knowledge. In these formulaic journal articles, methodology is not written or read as the perspectival text it is. (p. 122)

It is important to recognize that the intent of deconstructive analyses is not to unpack, unravel and in the process destroy everything and leave nothing in place. Nor is deconstruction anti-science or anti-method. It does not seek to reverse binaries in order to privilege yet another set of terms. In a deconstructive approach all terms are contested and are constantly open to scrutiny and challenge. Hence, deconstructive approaches expose deep assumptions and enable analyses that are able to be used to explore, contest and thereby possibly change, aspects of contemporary reality, including that of health care.

Finally, in rounding off this very brief introductory discussion of deconstruction, it is important not to give a sense of having provided "the" definition or understanding of deconstruction. All texts, including this one, are open to deconstruction: "every deconstruction can be deconstructed" (Agger 1991, p. 115). All authorial privilege is contested in order to expose the investments any author has made in the text they produce, including in research-based texts. What an author has put in and what they have left out reflects such investments. This is why Agger (1992) asserts that "deconstructive reading reads itself reading" (p. 95).

SUMMARY

Poststructural thought has much in common with postmodern perspectives. However, the focus of poststructural analysis is text, where the word "text" refers to a representation of any aspect of reality. The reality of the health care setting is mediated by texts which convey understandings of health care practice and in turn construct understandings themselves.

Discourse analysis is a useful approach to the interrogation of such texts. In discourse analysis, texts themselves, rather than the reality they purport to represent, are the data to be analyzed. How a text conveys certain understandings of the reality of health care is of as much interest as what that text conveys. Thus the analysis moves beyond the descriptive into the discursive.

Popular media represents health, disease and illness in certain ways and not in others. Discourse analysis enables an exploration of representations in terms of the way they are shaped by, and in turn shape, dominant discourses about health and health care.

Similarly, patients' case notes, a central feature of contemporary health care practice, can be explored using discourse analysis to reveal the way dominant understandings in health settings shape both the form and the content of those notes. Analysis of who or what is absent from the notes provides useful insights into other ways that practice can be represented and conceptualized.

Parker's (1992) features of discourse analysis provide a useful framework for studies involving discourse analysis. The section on discourse analysis ended by exploring some of the limitations of discourse analysis, particularly the concept of an active reader of texts—a reader who assumes a negotiated viewing or reading position with respect to the reading of any particular text.

Deconstruction, often associated with Derrida, is another approach drawing on poststructural thought. Agger's exploration of assumptions implicit within a deconstructive approach provides a useful introduction to deconstruction. The concept of binary oppositions gives important insights into what a deconstructive approach has to offer. Analyses of the way such oppositions work to create and sustain dominant understandings in the health care context are particularly useful. Finally, the way in which deconstruction troubles implicit assumptions and understandings about the research process itself is explored.

This concludes the first part of this book. In the chapters to follow, the discussion turns the focus from theoretical matters that have formed the basis of Chapters 1-3 to an exploration of more practical issues associated with these research approaches.

FURTHER READINGS

Agger, B. (1992). *Cultural studies as critical theory*. London: Falmer.

> Chapter 6, "Poststructuralism and Postmodernism on Culture", provides a description of the social and political context of deconstruction and of its relation to poststructural and postmodern thought. It also provides a comprehensive discussion on the features of a deconstructive reading of texts, identifying six features that form the basis of a deconstructive approach.

Cheek, J & Rudge, T. (1994b). Inquiry into nursing as textually mediated discourse. In P. Chinn (Ed.), *Advances in methods of inquiry for nursing* (pp. 59-67). Gaithserburg, MD: Aspen.

> This chapter describes discourse analysis and discusses the limitations of such an approach. It explores the notion of nursing as textually mediated, with reference to the research into case notes discussed in this chapter of this book.

Fox, N. (1995). Postmodern perspectives on care: The vigil and the gift. *Critical Sociology Today*, 15(2/3), 107-125.

> Fox explores the notion of binary oppositions through a discussion about two differing types of care, caring for and caring about. He seeks to develop the concept of care as a gift by shifting the focus away from aspects of care which focus on vigilance and domination toward those aspects of care which are devalued, such as generosity, trust and "being-with".

Lupton, D. (1992). Discourse analysis: A new methodology for understanding the ideologies of health and illness. *Australian Journal of Public Health*, 16(2), 145-150.

> Lupton explores two aspects of discourse analysis: the textual features which relate to the structure of the text and the contextual features, which relate the structural features to their social, political and cultural context. This concept of discourse analysis is explored in relation to public health research and with particular reference to media coverage of AIDS.

Parker, I. (1992). *Discourse dynamics: Critical analysis for social and individual psychology*. London: Routledge.

> Chapter 1, "Discovering Discourses, Tackling Texts" provides a comprehensive description of what discourse is and concludes with a brief discussion of Foucault's concept of discourse. Chapter 6, "Research and Reading" provides and elaborates on the steps for discourse analysis discussed in this text.

Weedon, C. (1987). *Feminist practice and post structuralist theory*. London: Basil Blackwell.

> Chapter 2, "Principles of Poststructuralism", discusses the centrality of language to poststructural thought in relation to some key poststructuralist theorists including Derrida. The chapter concludes with a discussion of Foucault's concept of discourse and of the discursive field. The discussion focuses on some of the dominant discourses surrounding women and of the power relations that attend these knowledges.

Chapter 4

Speaking Practically, Part 1:
"Proposing" Research Informed by Postmodern and Poststructural Approaches

OVERVIEW

The remaining chapters of this book discuss how to actually carry out research using postmodern and/or poststructural approaches. The previous chapters introduced (albeit briefly) postmodern and poststructural theoretical perspectives and demonstrated how these approaches, when applied in a research context, can inform aspects of nursing and health care practice. The discussion that follows assumes familiarity with the ideas presented earlier.

The first chapters of the book discussed in fairly general terms research projects carried out by various investigators. Invariably in these discussions the overall concept of the research was introduced, followed by a relatively small amount of detail about the way the research was carried out leading to a final discussion of the analysis of the findings. This is not dissimilar to the way research studies and findings are reported in the literature. Due to space constraints, and often due to conventions and understandings about what is or is not appropriate to report in scholarly articles, the finer detail about the research in question is left out. Thus, after reading such reports one often finds it hard to work out exactly what was done.

Rarely, if ever, are research proposals themselves published so that the conceptual development of the research project can be explored. Such invisibility of research proposals makes it difficult for less experienced and/or novice researchers in that they often find it hard to conceptualize what a research proposal using, for example, a postmodern approach might look like. It forces the beginning researcher to rely on obtaining proposals from more experienced researchers and/or having discussions with them, which may not always be possible.

We need to address the somewhat invisible nature of research proposals in the literature, and indeed even in research methods texts, so that much of this chapter revolves around a research proposal that I prepared for a particular funding agency and which was successful in gaining funding. Each part of the proposal will be examined and then discussed in terms of why it was written as it was. In this way the reader will have the advantage of seeing a proposal at the same time as having the reasons for the content and form of that proposal discussed. For these reasons the discussion will be grounded in the practical reality of writing proposals so that the proposal becomes the vehicle from which points about proposal writing can be generated. This is in contrast with the usual format in which general principles for proposal writing are identified and the assumption is made that the reader can go on to formulate proposals from such principles. It is important to note that the proposal being used is not being held up as an "ideal" or "perfect" proposal (as no such thing exists!). Rather, it is being used as an example of what a research proposal might look like. Each piece of proposed research will, of course, have its own emphasis and specific format. The form offering structure to the development of the proposal can be found in appendix A.

There will be another interesting twist at various points in this chapter as we examine the research proposal and the information it calls for using a postmodern/poststructural lens. Thus at times there are three levels of discussion operating at once:

- The content itself of the research proposal;
- How to meet the requirements of the funding body or other audience for whom the proposal is written; and
- The research proposal as an example of text and the unwritten and written rules and assumptions that shape it.

I hope that this will lead to lively, informative and in-depth analysis!

Having explored the development of the research proposal as well as what this exploration reveals about the craft of proposal writing, we will go on to examine the type of data collected when the proposed study was under way and the subsequent analysis of that data.

THE CRAFT OF PROPOSAL WRITING:
PRELIMINARY CONSIDERATIONS

Writing a research proposal is a craft. *The Macquarie Dictionary* (1985, p.102) offers the following definitions of craft:

> 1. skill; ingenuity; dexterity. 2. cunning; deceit; guile. 3. an art, trade, or occupation requiring special skill, esp. manual skill; a handicraft. 4. (construed as pl.) boats, ships, and vessels collectively.

It is the first and third definitions that are of interest to our discussion here. Crafting a well-constructed research proposal requires skill. It is an art and, like any art, it improves upon practice. Writing a research proposal also involves dexterity—the ability to "fit" and "tailor" a proposal to guides. It also requires both theoretical and methodological dexterity coupled with a touch of ingenuity to apply such theoretical and methodological frames to new or different substantive areas. It is hoped that no research proposal incorporates the elements of the second definition—cunning, deceit and guile!

I now wish to discuss some aspects of the art and skills needed in refining and writing research proposals. The first of these is writing for a particular audience. Consider who will read the proposal, how they will assess it, and how the proposal will need to be shaped in order to meet the expectations of that particular audience.

Writing for an Audience

Research proposals are examples of text. Like other texts such as journal articles, books, theses, medical reports and nursing notes they have a very specific form. As we have briefly discussed in Chapter 3 (see the section "Research as a text that can be deconstructed"), this form is shaped by certain dominant understandings of what an appropriate format for a research proposal is. As we have seen, arising from these dominant understandings are unwritten rules about what is (and thus what is not) appropriate subject matter for research, and what is (and thus what is not) a suitable way of carrying out the research.

For example, if the application instructions/guidelines for a research grant insist that a hypothesis be given, then the unwritten assumption in operation is that all research should conform to the form demanded by the scientific method. It effectively excludes other types of research for which hypotheses are not relevant. A discourse analysis or a deconstruction study will not conform to such assumptions, nor will research that is designed to be exploratory and/or descriptive. The researcher who wishes to use research approaches for which hypotheses are not appropriate is left in a situation in which their research does not "fit" the assumed form for a research proposal. It is important to recognize that this does not mean that research which does not "fit" such assumptions is alternative and somehow less valuable. Rather, such research does not conform to one set of understandings about what research might be and what it might involve, or concomitantly to assumptions about how knowledge develops.

Along with such unwritten rules are written rules in the guidelines to filling in research application forms which specify the format an application will take. These may include what should be discussed, how much is required to be discussed (i.e., length of each section), and by default, what does not need to be stated. These rules "force" researchers to adopt the specified format. To not do so would inevitably result in the application being assessed as incomplete and consequently not able to be funded. Table 4.1 gives an example of such rules in action.

TABLE 4.1: Guidelines for the Preparation of a Small Australian Research Council Grants for 1996.

Aims, research plan, justification of budget, and publications

---

To answer this question fully, you may wish to refer to the "Guidelines for 1996 ARC Large Research Grants" so that you can cover the points specifically made in it, especially in relation to policy and priority information and detailed justification of the budget proposal. A copy of these guidelines is available from the Research Office.

Your explanation should be comprehensive but brief.

No more than 13 pages, including this form (but excluding publications), will be considered in the assessment process.

Pages in excess will be discarded.

Use the following headings to detail your answer:

* Aims and significance
* Research plan, methods and techniques
* Progress Report, where project has already commenced
* Justification of Budget
* Timetable
* Benefits of research
* Plans to apply for external funds to continue the project (Research Development Grant only)
* Publications—you should list all your refereed publications for the last 5 years. Use asterisks to identify publications relevant to this project.

Where the cooperation or assistance of another body is needed for the project to be successful, the Grants Sub-Committee must be provided with appropriate details.

This brings me to the first point that I want to make about the craft of proposal writing. All proposals for research are written for particular audiences. Types of audiences may include funding bodies, ethics committees and, if the proposal forms part of a student's program of study, course review committees. Each audience has its own expectations—its own written and unwritten rules for how the proposal should be framed. Thus, it is important to know your audience and to assess its expectations. This is particularly useful with respect to funding bodies. Some funding bodies will only fund certain types of research, whereas others may be more open to a range of approaches. If a postmodern or poststructural approach is to form part of a proposed piece of research, it is important to ascertain that the audience who will be reviewing the proposal is amenable or open to considering that research approach.

It is also important to consider whether the outcomes of the research will be of interest to the proposal's audience. For example, a course review team might consider a theoretical treatise on some aspect of health care a perfectly reasonable research outcome whereas a funding body concerned with developing cost-efficient modes of health care delivery may be less likely to see the value in that outcome.

Research proposal writing is, at least to some extent, a political process. It is important to be aware of the expectations and assumptions (both spoken and unspoken) of the audience for whom you are writing. Choose the body from which you wish to apply for funding carefully. Consider if the approach to research you wish to take and the outcomes you are proposing fit with the agenda of that funding body. If they do not, then it is unlikely that you will be successful in your application. Search for an audience that seems amenable to the approach you are suggesting.

Meanwhile, there is nothing to stop you from writing to funding bodies that seem closed to the approaches you are suggesting and pointing out the difficulty that their application guidelines/instructions pose for certain types of research. My own experience has demonstrated that sometimes funding agencies do not realize how restrictive the guidelines they have developed are for health research that does not fit the scientific/medical model. It is possible to agitate for change. I have found myself invited to address funding panels to discuss the issues I had raised in a letter, and in one instance I ended up assisting in the revision of the application form and guidelines so that they became more inclusive of different approaches to research. Researching the audience for whom you are writing is thus, in some ways, of as much importance as the development of the actual research proposal itself!

Formulating a Question

Another important skill in the craft of proposal writing is the ability to formulate a clear, precise and feasible research question. Indeed, the first step in formulating any research proposal is deciding exactly what it is that will be studied. What is the issue/question/problem/hypothesis that will be the focus of the study? As we have seen, whether what you develop is an issue, a question, a problem or an hypothesis is an integral part of formulating the research question and consequently formulating the approach to the research that will be taken. Ideas for research can arise from issues you confront in your everyday life, in your professional role, in what you have read in both professional and popular literature such as magazines and newspapers, in conversations with others, or in formal courses of study.

Regardless of the source of the initial inspiration for the research topic/area, the development of the idea into a proposal will involve considerations of the theoretical orientation and methodology to be employed in the study. This will necessarily lead you to consider what type of data you will collect and the reasons for collecting that data. The type of material or data collected in a study will depend on the theoretical and methodological frames employed.

However, no matter what these frames might be, even if they are postmodern or poststructural approaches, there are certain criteria that can be used to distinguish what Schutt (1996) terms:

> good research questions from mediocre ones. A good research question will be *feasible* within the time and resources available, it will be *socially important*, and it will be *scientifically relevant.* (p. 35)

What Schutt tells us is that a good research question will build on and add to existing knowledge in the particular substantive area that is the focus of the research.

Developing a question, topic or issue into a researchable form takes times and energy. No doubt the research concept will undergo considerable refinement from the time it is first thought of to the moment it appears in text in the form of a written research proposal. The bodies of literature developed about particular issues/topics and substantive areas provide valuable assistance in refining the research topic. The literature can be used to reveal what other studies have been done in this area, what research techniques have been used, and whether or not your proposed research seems feasible.Later in this chapter we will explore in more detail the role of the literature in formulating a research proposal. Once your question has been refined, it is possible to establish aims for the study and your methods for researching the particular area. However, until you have clearly refined the question or issue that drives your research, you will not be able to move any further in your proposal development. As simple as it may sound, identifying and formulating a question for the research is a complex skill integral to the craft of proposal writing.

Establishing the Credentials of Both the Research and the Researcher

Another important skill pertaining to the craft of developing a research proposal is that of "selling" the research and the researcher(s). It is essential that you neither undersell yourself nor overstate your expertise. The skill lies in giving a honest account of the credentials of both the researcher(s) and the proposed research.

The information requested in the first part of a proposal is used to contextualize both the research and the researcher. Thus, the name(s) of the chief investigator(s) will be called for early on. This information indicates who will work on the project and what role and what responsibilities each person will have if there is more than one researcher on the project. This information will be used to establish the credentials and expertise of the researcher or the research team. Such credentials and expertise are determined by reference to the named chief investigator's track record. Track record is usually established in terms of other grant monies won and publications (such as refereed articles, book chapters or books). It is important to provide clear and complete information that is easy to follow. Grants and publications should be listed from the most recent to the least recent. All names of investigators for the grants or authors of the publications should be given.

In the list of grants and publications, I have found it useful to bold the names of the investigator(s) for the grant being applied for so that it is easy for reviewers assessing the grant to see the relevant name(s), especially if they are part of a team of authors or grant recipients. For example, the list might read:

> **Cheek, J**. (Principal Investigator), Ruffin, R., & Pincombe, J. $71,524.00 gained from the PHARM Scheme, Pharmaceutical Benefits Branch of the Department of Health Housing, Local Government and Community Services, for the project "Knowing What Needs to be Known: A Consumer Asthma Medication Study".

> **Cheek, J.**, & Gibson, T. (1997). Policy matters: Critical policy analysis and nursing. *Journal of Advanced Nursing*, 25, 668-672.

> Lange, A. & **Cheek, J.** (1997). Health policy and the nursing profession—A deafening silence. *International Journal of Nursing Practice, 3*, 2-9.

Neither an individual's practical experience in a particular area or his or her oral conference presentations are usually afforded as much standing as published papers when establishing and evaluating an individual's track record. Often the instructions limit the listing to certain publications and types of grants, or there is simply no space provided to list practical experience credentials or conference presentations. Establishing credentials in research draws on often taken-for-granted understandings of either what does or does not "count" in terms of track record or how much each aspect does count in relative terms. The written word (and particularly certain types of written word) is afforded primacy over the spoken word. There is a binary opposition (see Chapter 3, the section "The concept of binary oppositions") in operation here.

At the same time as the researcher(s) is being situated in terms of credentials, the research itself is contextualized. A title, and often keywords, are requested so that the proposed research can be situated. A short summary or synopsis is required to provide an overview of the project in a clear, stand-alone manner that describes the context, objectives, methods and likely benefits of the project. Information is requested about whether ethics approval is necessary for the research, and if so whether it has been gained or is being sought. Funding is usually dependent on ethical approval being gained before the money is received. Although it is beyond the scope of this chapter to discuss in anything but a passing manner the considerations regarding the ethics of any piece of research, even research from postmodern and poststructural approaches, such considerations include:

–   Confidentiality of participants and data

–   Safety of participants

–   Value as opposed to risks of the research

–   Data handling and storage

–   Informed consent of participants
–   Right of participants to withdraw from the study at any time

Finally, in terms of contextualizing the research, applicants are often required to state the benefits or outcomes of the research. This can determine whether the research is worthwhile. However, as we have seen, "worthwhile" may mean different things to different people and to different funding audiences. Depending on the intended audience of the proposal, the benefits of research might pertain to economic benefits such as reduction of costs of delivery or service provision in health care; social benefits such as increase in quality of life; policy benefits; institutional or organizational benefits; or any other type of benefit.

The following excerpt is the "benefits" section of a proposal for an Australian Research Council (ARC) small grant. These grants are awarded through universities by the ARC for high quality research projects and pilot research projects of modest cost conducted by researchers of proven excellence. A secondary objective is to support new researchers who show clear evidence of high research capacity. Funding is provided in the social sciences for amounts of up to $19,999.

When reading the following "benefits" section can you determine the audience I was writing for?

> The benefit of this research lies in its potential to uncover the way in which Toxic Shock Syndrome has been represented in 4 examples of Australian print based media, including the often overlooked popular magazine genre, in order to explore the impact that such representation has on the construction of understandings of Toxic Shock Syndrome, tampon use, menstruation and women's health more generally. It will reveal the vested interests that may be present in the reporting of Toxic Shock Syndrome, especially in terms of whether it is a tampon related/induced health risk. Once such representation is analysed and its effects better understood it will be possible to design relevant health promotion strategies and information packages for women pertaining to Toxic Shock Syndrome, the use of tampons and other related health issues.

The benefits I identified as being derived from this research fit into several categories:

–   Contribution to new knowledge about the way health and illness are represented in popular print-based media—a benefit directly related to the generation of knowledge and scholarship
–   Examination of competing interests in the portrayals of health and illness—a political analysis
–   Practical outcomes derived from the research which can assist health promotion and the development of health information—benefits directly related to the delivery of health care and to the provision of health-related information

Thus, if I have targeted an appropriate funding audience, the ARC is likely to be a body which is interested in both the generation of new knowledge by research and practical outcomes derived from research. Indeed, it is precisely these areas which are evident in the five benefits of research that the ARC itself identifies. The guidelines ask researchers to identify one or more of these benefits to which the proposed research relates. The five benefits stated by the ARC are:

– Contribution to the quality of our culture
– Graduates of high quality
– Direct application of research results
– Increased institutional capacity for consulting, contract research and other services
– International links

The proposed project about toxic shock syndrome relates to two of the five benefits of research specified namely:

1. Contributions to the quality of our culture in that the project enables an Australian perspective on world wide scholarly debate about the representations of health and illness. It does so in a unique way, using sources of material that are somewhat taken for granted. The impact of popular women's magazines on particular cultural understandings in Australia (and indeed world wide) has been relatively neglected.

2. Direct applications of research results. The project will facilitate, by analysis of the way toxic shock syndrome is represented, the design of relevant health promotion strategies and information packages pertaining to toxic shock syndrome, the use of tampons and other related health issues for both consumers and health professionals.

Finally, it should not surprise you to find an emphasis on an Australian perspective in this research as the funding body is the Australian Research Council.

THE CRAFT OF PROPOSAL WRITING: CREATING THE TEXT

The previous section has indicated some of the more preliminary considerations that form part of any skilled development of a research proposal. These considerations are pertinent to proposals that outline research using postmodern and poststructural approaches. In particular, it is crucial to consider the audience for the proposal. I now wish to focus the discussion on writing a research proposal using postmodern and poststructural frames. This moves the level of discussion to the practical task of capturing the proposed research in written form whilst conforming to prescribed space and content criteria.

As stated previously, many research textbooks discuss the various sections of "standard" research proposals such as the aims and background without demonstrating what such a section may look like in an actual proposal.

The following discussion of crafting a research proposal takes a different approach. Sections of a research proposal are used to highlight the points being made about the skills needed to develop research proposals. The research proposal used is one I submitted to the Australian Research Council (ARC) Small Grants Scheme. We have already begun to examine this proposal in the discussion about benefits of research in a previous section of this chapter.

The guidelines and application form for the ARC Small Grants are fairly standard in terms of the layout and of the categories of information requested. Therefore, it should be possible for you to extrapolate the discussion and points made here to other application forms and guidelines that may vary slightly from the example here. It is the principles involved in the craft of proposal writing which are the focus of our exploration and we will use the examples cited to identify these principles.

The title of the research project outlined in the proposal to the ARC Small Grants Scheme was "Constructing Toxic Shock Syndrome: Selected print-based media representations of Toxic Shock Syndrome from 1979-1995". I will contextualize the research for you the reader in the same way as I did for the funding body, by providing you with the synopsis of the proposed research:

> The way in which the print based media, including popular magazines, represents health issues, influences and shapes societal attitudes towards illness and understandings of health risk. This study explores the way in which a relatively new health phenomenon, Toxic Shock Syndrome, has been represented in Australian print based media from 1979-1995. In so doing it will, by textual analysis of articles pertaining to Toxic Shock Syndrome, uncover changing and different representations of Toxic Shock Syndrome and their effect on perceptions of Toxic Shock Syndrome and related women's health issues and risks.

This synopsis outlines in broad terms, using non-technical and jargon-free language, what the proposed research is about. The synopsis is important as it is often used to locate the research in terms of which assessment panel and/or expert referees it should go to for evaluation and comment. When funding bodies receive proposals initially, the proposals are often sorted on the basis of their substantive and/or methodological focus. The grants are then sent to those individuals considered to have an understanding of the approach used in the proposal and of the area in which the research is located substantively. Such "experts" may form a panel to adjudicate grants themselves. More often, the panel will do an initial cull of grants on the basis of general criteria such as completeness of proposal, readability, worth and so forth, and then send surviving applications out to review by independent, anonymous referees for comment. Thus it is absolutely critical that the synopsis and any key words that might be given convey an adequate sense of what the research is about and the approach taken so that a good match is obtained between the research proposed and the understandings and expertise of those who assess it.

Furthermore, if it is not possible to outline in clear, everyday language what the research proposal is about then the clarity of the entire research project is bought into question. I quite often leave the writing of the synopsis or summary of the research until I have completed writing the proposal. This is to ensure that the summary is an accurate reflection of what is actually proposed. Proposals evolve, and it is important that synopses are indicative of the final proposal rather than of the earlier stages of proposal development!

We now need to consider the various sections of a research proposal and how they might be crafted.

Aims

Like any piece of research, research emanating from postmodern and/or poststructural approaches must have clear aims and objectives. The aims for the project under discussion were as follows:

The project will

1   Locate articles relating to Toxic Shock Syndrome appearing in selected Australian print based media between 1979-1995.

2   Use descriptive statistics to build a longitudinal picture of the extent, timing (month/year) and type of reporting of issues concerning Toxic Shock Syndrome in these media.

3   Analyse the content of the reporting to ascertain prevalent themes evident in such reporting.

4   Explore the discourses present about Toxic Shock Syndrome in the articles found, thereby exploring ways in which these print based media create and sustain understandings of Toxic Shock Syndrome, menstruation and women's health.

5   Provide the basis for better understanding of the discursive construction by print based media of Toxic Shock Syndrome specifically, and women's health generally, in order to ensure appropriate targeting of further research into representations of Toxic Shock Syndrome and to allow for the development of more appropriate and relevant educational programs and information material for women with respect to Toxic Shock Syndrome, menstruation, tampon use and other related health issues.

These aims are very clear. They tell the reader exactly what the study hopes to achieve at each phase of the project. Further, they clearly locate the study theoretically by referring to discourse and discursive construction. The final aim indicates what the investigator hopes to achieve in terms of practical implications and applications for health care practice. Once they have been established, the aims of the study guide the development of the rest of the proposal. All material incorporated into the proposal must clearly relate to the stated aims.

Background and Significance

In this section of the proposal, which sometimes can be called "critical literature review", the "why" question is answered with respect to the research being proposed. Why is this research important? Why does it need to be done? How does it fit with other work and studies that have been done in the area?

In other words, this section of the proposal contextualizes the research in terms of what has gone before. It should demonstrate the researcher's understanding of a particular area. It should also demonstrate that there is a need for the research being proposed and that the research has not been done before. Often there are strict space constraints on this section, so selectivity is needed in terms of what is or is not included. Any key or core studies in the area should be cited, including those studies which may have indicated a need for this research to be done. It is important that the background and significance of the project clearly relates to the aims and objectives identified in the proposal.

The following excerpt is the background and significance section from the Small ARC research proposal. It is reasonably lengthy, but you may want to read it with the following points in mind. Does this excerpt:

- Indicate why the proposed research is important?
- Explain how it fits with other work and studies done in the area?
- Cite key works in the area?

If so, do the cited studies:

- Indicate the need for research such as that proposed here?
- Provide information which clearly relates to the aims of the study?

You may also want to think about how this section is structured. How does it begin? How does it establish both the theoretical and substantive frames to be employed in the study? Finally, how does the discussion turn to focus on the expected outcomes and benefits of the research? Considering questions such as these will give you insights into the craft of proposal construction. You may want to make notes in the margins to assist your analysis. Such analysis can provide you with a structural frame around which you can build the background and significance sections for proposals you may write. The background and significance section of the proposal read as follows:

> *Much of the current research into health and illness asserts that many diseases are not value free, scientific entities. Instead, it is apparent that the manner in which certain diseases are represented in social texts, such as the press or magazines, is influenced by societal beliefs and values (Fox 1993b; Lupton 1994c, 1994d, 1995).*

Furthermore, such research reveals that the way diseases or health are represented may hide assumptions which underpin the very definitions of health and illness themselves. An outcome of this work is that understandings of health, illness, and disease processes cannot be viewed as independent of the social context in which they are situated.

Lupton (1995) asserts that the news media is one of the most important contemporary forums for the articulation of discourses, that is, particular ways of thinking and talking about reality (Foucault 1980), relating to health and medicine. "A discourse provides a set of possible statements about a given area, and organises and gives structure to the manner in which a particular topic, object, process is to be talked about" (Kress 1985, p.7). Who is quoted, who is not; what sources are used and how an article is framed affects perceptions of the health issue being reported. News is thus a representation of a particular view of reality, not a value-free reflection of facts. "All news is always reported from some particular angle" (Fowler 1991, p.10).

For example, Gabe, Gustafsson and Bury (1991) analysed the content of newspaper coverage on the issue of women's tranquilliser dependence. Their analysis highlighted the importance of taking into account ways in which mass communication can distort and bias understandings about dependence, how it can reaffirm stereotypical understandings about women's passivity, and how it can thereby conceal crucial difference between groups or individuals who are dependent on tranquillisers. Chrisler and Levy (1990) found, on analysis of media content on Pre-menstrual Syndrome (PMS), that the messages conveyed by the media confused biologically based premenstrual changes with the actual syndrome, so that PMS became so inclusive in focus that it would be difficult for women not to find at least part of their experience recorded. Further, Stallings (1990) has demonstrated that perception of health risk is not so much the outcome of media and public discourse as existing in and through processes of that discourse. "Hence risk is never constant. It is created and recreated in discussion of events that are seen to undermine a world taken for granted" (p. 82).

Likewise, articles and reporting in popular magazines, a largely overlooked area, reflect certain representations of reality. Baird and Sheridan's (1992) analysis of the Australian Women's Weekly leads them to assert with respect to developing an index for the popular women's magazine, "the most interesting feature of the construction of the index thus far has been the insight into the reader positions that the Weekly constructs" (p.150).

Albert's (1986) study of how a sample of nationally circulated magazines in the US treated and represented a new medical phenomenon—AIDS— clearly demonstrated the effect of this genre of print based media in creating certain understandings and perceptions of AIDS.

Studies such as these alert researchers to the need to consider the role of media representations themselves in constructing images of health/illness, and the social understandings of health/illness that result from such representations. As Nelkin (1991) asserts, newspapers and popular magazines:

> filled with health advisory columns, as well as news about risk events, dominate the avenues of public information....The information they convey, their visual and verbal images, and tone of the presentation can define the significance of events, shape public attitudes and legitimate or call into question public policies. (p.302)

This is true of the reporting about Toxic Shock Syndrome.

Toxic Shock Syndrome (TSS) was first named as such in 1978 by James K. Todd (Hanrahan 1994) in Denver, USA. However, it possibly has been present in the medical literature since 1927 usually described as staphylococcal scarlet fever (Colbry 1992). Toxic Shock Syndrome symptoms include the sudden onset of high fever, vomiting, shock, body rash and peeling skin. Toxic Shock Syndrome's specific causative agent is the bacterium staphylococcus aureus. Whilst the majority of Toxic Shock Syndrome patients are menstruating women; non-menstruating women, children and men have contracted Toxic Shock Syndrome. Toxic Shock Syndrome has been linked to tampon use during menstruation but the exact nature of the linkage between tampons, the bacterium and Toxic Shock Syndrome remains problematic. The link between Toxic Shock Syndrome and tampon use was first reported in mid 1979 and early 1980 when Toxic Shock Syndrome resulted in the hospitalisation of 7 people in Wisconsin, USA—6 of whom were menstruating women using high absorbency tampons and one of whom was male (Olesen 1986). This led to massive media coverage and the subsequent construction of Toxic Shock Syndrome as an emergent new health risk. How the media reported on, and thus constructed understandings of Toxic Shock Syndrome from its discovery in 1978 up until the present (end of 1995) is the focus of this study.

Discourses surrounding Toxic Shock Syndrome are particularly problematic as Toxic Shock Syndrome touches on taboo areas such as menstruation and sanitary products (Delaney, Lupton & Toth 1988).

Further, there are competing and vested interests in portrayals of Toxic Shock Syndrome such as those of tampon manufacturers, health authorities, consumer groups and so on. As Olesen declares:

the toxic shock phenomenon poses critical questions in the definition and construction of the issues ... certainly in the case of toxic shock syndrome, different definitions, predicated on the production of research data and the presumed confounding influences of the mass media of communication were and remain in play (1986, pp. 57-8).

Indeed, in a recent edition of the Australian Medical Journal, Garland and Peel (1995) declare Australians have been subjected to misleading information about Toxic Shock Syndrome in media publicity about the recent death of a girl in Queensland.

This study aims to address the question of the way in which Toxic Shock Syndrome has been defined and constructed as a health issue, since its formal recognition in 1978 and link to tampon use in 1979. It will provide a systematic overview of some of the Australian print based media reporting that has been done about Toxic Shock Syndrome in order to explore how Toxic Shock Syndrome has been constructed and what interests have been represented in that construction. Such analysis is essential if effects of the reporting, especially with respect to Toxic Shock Syndrome as a public health issue, are to be exposed and understood. Only then can moves be made to reveal Toxic Shock Syndrome from all angles—not just those constructed by certain media. This is imperative as "the media provide and reflect blueprints for action" (Clarke 1991, p.304). The significance of the study thus lies in attempting to answer (at least in part) Clarke's question "if the media reflect biased views of disease, its causes, meanings and best treatment alternatives, what can be done to ensure more appropriate portrayals?" (1991, p.305). Timely and responsible reporting is critically important to the management of Toxic Shock Syndrome (Colbry 1992).

How did your analysis and exploration of the way in which this section has been crafted go? Were you able to identify the structural framework underpinning this section? Points to note about such a framework include (and you may find it useful to mark the sections of the background and significance section that pertain to each of the points made in order to get a "visual" sense of how this section was constructed):

– The section begins at a macro theoretical level. It discusses textual representations of disease and illness and posits that any such representation conceals assumptions and understandings about the definitions of health and illness

–   Having established the broad theoretical frame, the discussion moves "down" one theoretical level to look at the way two types of texts—news media and popular magazines—have represented aspects of health care practice and health care reality. Studies are cited for each type of text, and these studies are used to demonstrate the possibilities for analysis of health issues afforded by exploring the way these texts portray and represent disease and illness

–   This opening part, which contextualizes the research theoretically and in terms of studies that have been done in the area, ends by asserting the importance of the type of study proposed, arguing from Nelkin (1991) that such representation can "define the significance of events, shape public attitudes and legitimate—or call into question—public policies" (p. 302)

–   The discussion then turns to look at the particular health topic that will form the substantive focus of the proposed research. After describing Toxic Shock Syndrome (TSS), the research is brought into clear focus at the end of the introductory discussion about TSS with the statement: "How the media reported on, and thus constructed understandings of Toxic Shock Syndrome from its discovery in 1978 up until the present (end of 1995) is the focus of this study". This statement relates clearly to the stated aims of the project. Thus there is already congruence between the various sections of the proposal. Such congruence is an essential part of the craft of proposal writing

–   The discussion then turns to introduce the notion of discourses that shape the way TSS is written, spoken and thought about

–   In terms of setting the scene for the background and significance of the study, the discussion returns to the aims of the study and discusses how these fit with the concepts and ideas that have arisen in the background section

–   The last point in this section reinforces the significance of the study and relates it to health care practice.

In summary, the background and significance section locates the study in a theoretical sense, where such "location" may operate at various levels of theoretical analysis. It then links the theoretical frame of the study to the substantive area under discussion and demonstrates how the theoretical approach taken can lead to new and important insights into the area under discussion. In so doing, it refers to other studies that can illuminate aspects of the proposed research. Finally, the discussion clearly articulates the aims of the study. It emphasizes the significance of the study in terms of its implications for, and application to, the field of research (in this case health care delivery, practice and understandings).

Research Plan, Methods and Techniques

Having established the "why" and "what" in relation to the proposed research, a proposal will then need to outline the "how". How will the research be carried out? It is important that the research plan be congruent with the theoretical orientation of the study and with its stated aims. One of the issues that confronts researchers when writing this section of the proposal is how much detail to include about the methods themselves and the actual analytic techniques.

A good starting point when grappling with this issue is to look at how much space the application guide or form allows for each section. If it stipulates one page only, for example, then much less detail can be given than if three to four pages are allowed. Another issue to consider is whether some terms could reasonably be expected to be understood by reviewers. Determining this is not easy, but the type of funding scheme may give you a clue. For example, if you are writing an application in a granting scheme that has traditionally funded empirical, scientific research then you will need to give clear explanations of terms and ideas that may be unfamiliar to the reviewers and/or panel of this scheme. If, on the other hand, you are applying to a funding body that has funded research using postmodern and/or poststructural approaches in the past, then it may not be as necessary to go into as much conceptual detail. However, there are no hard and fast rules about what detail and what level of that detail to include in an application. As well as doing my homework about the funding scheme I intend to apply for, as outlined previously, another strategy I have found useful is to examine copies of successful grant applications in the particular scheme I am interested in. Reading these applications will give a sense of what level of detail is appropriate.

We will now look at writing the research plan, methods and techniques section of a proposal by exploring this section of the grant proposal.. As you read it, ask yourself the following questions:

- Does the methodology "fit" with the theoretical orientation of the study?
- Is there a clear link with the aims of the project?
- Will the research plan outlined enable the researcher to achieve the aims?
- Is the proposed research feasible?

Methodology

The study comprises an exploratory critical analysis (see Lupton 1994c) of the reporting of issues associated with Toxic Shock Syndrome in selected Australian print media from 1979-1995. In so doing it incorporates traditional content analysis studies of media (Bell, Boehringer & Crofts 1982; Winston 1990). However, the focus does not rest only on the manifest (Lupton 1994c) or surface content as many traditional content analyses do.

Instead the study seeks to probe the latent or subtextual (Lupton 1994c) discourses (Foucault 1977) that both construct and are constructed, about Toxic Shock Syndrome.

The methodology section draws on concepts presented in the background/significance section of the proposal. The methods section goes on to give specific detail as to how this will actually be done.

Methods

Working within the framework of critical analysis, the study will survey and locate all articles pertaining to Toxic Shock Syndrome appearing in 4 purposively selected (after Clarke 1991) print based Australian media from 1979-end of 1995. 1979 has been chosen as a starting point for the study as Todd identified Toxic Shock Syndrome in late 1978. The sample is purposive in that the 4 print based media have been chosen to reflect diverse Australian target audiences thus providing a potentially rich supply of data in terms of the angle from which each reports and constructs Toxic Shock Syndrome.

The print based media to be surveyed comprise:

1. The Australian Women's Weekly

A once weekly, now monthly, women's popular magazine with a circulation (1995) of 1 million and estimated readership of 3.4 million, chosen because of its long standing place in Australian culture as a women's magazine of broad appeal. As McNicoll (1982, p.40) puts it, "almost everyone at some time or other has read it...its appeal crossing the barriers of the sexes, a magazine aimed at women but finishing up with a unisex appeal".

2. Cleo

A monthly Women's Lifestyle magazine with a circulation (December 1994) of 328,329 chosen because it was developed to address the new woman of the 1970s "liberated, active and outspoken" (Craik 1989, p.38) and targets women of age 20-40 years.

3. Dolly

A monthly teenage girl's magazine with a circulation of 167,000 in 1995 and estimated readership of 637,000. First released in 1970— "the first magazine of its kind in Australia insofar as it appeals specifically to a group hitherto not targeted by the mass media, adolescent girls" (Bail, Murray-Smith & Shaw 1985, p.85).

4. The Advertiser

A daily (Monday-Saturday) state broadsheet with circulation of 203,116 on weekdays and 265,583 on Saturdays and an estimated readership of 603,000 on weekdays and 734,000 on Saturdays. As the only daily state based newspaper in South Australia since March 1992, it is highly influential in informing views and constructing understandings of issues in South Australia.

Method of Locating Articles

1. The Australian Women's Weekly

This magazine is not indexed, so a manual search is the best option for locating articles. Back issues are held by the Flinders University Main Library on microfilm from the first issue (June 1933) up until 1983. The South Australian State Library (Mortlock) holds issues on microfilm until December 1994, and hard copies for 1995 (active subscription). Photocopies may be obtained of any articles. Photocopying is cheaper from Flinders University so articles up until 1983 will be obtained from there, and subsequently from Mortlock Library.

2. Cleo

This magazine is not indexed, so again a manual search in order to locate articles will be necessary. The State Library (Mortlock) holds Cleo issues from January 1979 to January 1990 on microfilm. The Cleo Magazine hold issues from the first issue until the present, and have agreed to photocopy the contents pages from February 1990 to end of 1995 and forward them. From the contents pages, it will be possible to select articles/letters/other items of interest and order further photocopies either from the publishers or the Australian National Library.

3. Dolly

This magazine is not indexed, so again a manual search is necessary. No library in South Australia has back copies from as far back as 1979, however, Dolly Magazine has agreed to photocopy the Contents pages from January 1979 until 1995 and forward them. From the contents pages it will be possible to select articles/letters/other items of interest and obtain photocopies of the articles from them.

4. The Advertiser

From 1986 until 1995, articles will be located using PRESSCOM, a data/indexing base which is updated daily and covers local, national and international news-gathering sources. Full text articles from 1986, including in-depth reports, Letters to the Editor, finance, sport, and general news are available for searching. Prior to 1986, however,-a manual search is required. The Advertiser is held at the Barr Smith Library on microfilm from 1858 until June 1995, and on hard copy until the present (active subscription).

Analysis of the Articles

Having obtained the articles a triangulation (Denzin 1989) of methods will be used in the analysis in order to provide a "thick description" (Denzin 1989). Such triangulation involves 3 phases of analysis:

Phase 1. Each article obtained will be analysed in terms of:
a)   *Headline*
b)   *Topic*
c)   *Visual material*
d)   *Sources quoted*
e)   *Whether it is primarily theoretical or practical*
f)   *Tone—positive or negative?*
g)   *Position in paper/magazine*
h)   *Relationship (if any) to other news articles at the time*
i)   *Type of print media it appears in*
j)   *Type of audience article pitched at*
k)   *Day of week*
l)   *Month of year*
m)   *Year*

Descriptive statistics will be applied to the above categories in order to build a picture of the extent, range, location, timing and type of reporting of issues concerning Toxic Shock Syndrome in these media. This draws on categories of analysis from studies by Lupton (1994a)—categories a, b, c & d; Gabe, Gustafsson and Bury (1991)—categories i & j; and Chrisler and Levy (1990) categories e and f. Additional categories (g, h, k, l & m) will further describe the construction of Toxic Shock Syndrome as a health issue from 1979-1995.

Phase 2. Qualitative thematic analysis of the articles will be employed in this phase.

The actual text of each article will be thematically coded then analysed. Both manifest and latent content will be themed.

Phase 3. The data obtained from Phase 1 and Phase 2 will be used to explore the discourses present about Toxic Shock Syndrome in order to develop an analysis of the representation of this health issue. This paves the way for further studies such as the effect on women of the way Toxic Shock Syndrome is represented in the media; and their understandings of Toxic Shock Syndrome, menstruation, tampon use, and other related health issues. Further, an interesting study could be done on Australian media representations of Toxic Shock Syndrome as opposed to, say, those in the US. A limitation of this study is that is restricted to 4 print based media only. A larger study could analyse more print based media sources.

Having read the excerpt, let us return to the questions posed at the outset of this section and consider each in turn. Does the methodology "fit" with the theoretical orientation of the study? The theoretical orientation of the study problematizes the representation of health and illness by print-based media, arguing that such representations reflect certain understandings of health/illness and conceal others. Thus the methodology employed should enable the way representations of health/illness are discursively constructed to be explored. As an exploratory critical analysis the study enables such analysis.

Is there a clear link with the aims? Yes, there is! In fact, if you look closely at the structure of the "methods" section you will notice that it is framed around the aims of the study. For example, the section clearly outlines what articles will be located and how this will be done (see aim 1 in the earlier section "Aims"). It also contains a clear statement about why these particular media were chosen (a purposive sample) which is very important in terms of the research design. A substantial amount of detail is given about the methods for locating the articles as it is important to establish the feasibility of the study, whether the articles can in fact be obtained, and what are the likely costs associated with locating them (discussed in the budget section of the proposal later). The methods section then moves on to address how each article will be analyzed: descriptively in Phase 1 of the analysis and thematically in Phase 2. This directly relates to Aims 2 and 3 of the study. Finally, Phase 3 of the research plan outlines the discursive phase of the analysis, which relates to Aim 4.

Thus not only have clear links been made to the aims of the study but the aims have in fact provided the framework around which the discussion in the methods section has been structured. Hence the third question posed at the outset of this section (Will the research plan outlined enable the researcher to achieve the aims?) has also been answered. As there is congruence between the aims and the proposed methods, the research plan should enable the aims to be met.

Finally, the level of detail provided in the methods section clearly demonstrates the feasibility of what is being proposed and the extent to which the researcher has thought the research process through. These are both very important. The research plan must be precise, concise, and above all, manageable. There is a somewhat deceptive simplicity in good research design.

Thus, in summary, the methodology section clearly situates this research in terms of other studies which the proposed research design, at least in part, emulated. Having outlined the overarching methodological frame, it went on to outline specific methods for collecting the research materials, including a rationale for the four print-based media chosen for the study. At all times there was a clear link between the methods being proposed and the aims of the study. The feasibility of the proposal was addressed in the detail provided about the location of each magazine/newspaper and in the way in which articles would be accessed. This is important, as otherwise it may have been difficult to assess whether what was being proposed could in fact be done!

Having established the mechanics of collecting the articles, the proposal outlined the way in which the articles would be analyzed. Again you will notice that appropriate reference was made to other studies. The source of the research material should be very clear to the reader of a proposal as should the weays in which it is going to be analyzed. This applies to research using postmodern and poststructural approaches just as it does to any other approach to research.

Timetable and Budget

Other sections of the proposal to be addressed are the time frame/time line for the research and the budget. The latter should include a justification for each of the budget items requested, while both the budget and the time frame should relate clearly to the rest of the proposal. For example, the time frame for the grant about Toxic Shock Syndrome read as follows:

Timetable
Months from Receipt of Grant

1-4: Phase 1

Location and collection of articles (see. aim 1). Progressive entry of descriptive statistics as per Phase 1 in Research Plan (see aim 2).

Completion of phase 1

5-9: Phase 2

Qualitative thematic analysis of articles and coding s per Phase 2 in Research Plan (see aim 3).

Completion phase 2

10-12 : Phase 3

Exploration of discursive construction of Toxic Shock Syndrome and analysis of possible effects on women's understandings of Toxic Shock Syndrome and associated health issues as per Phase 3 in Research Plan (see aim 4).

Completion and production of final report (see aim 5).

Report submitted to ARC, University of South Australia and any other interested parties.

Here the proposed sequence and timing of the research clearly articulates with the phases outlined in the research plan and the aims of the project. Similarly, the budget for the project is given in Table 4.2.

TABLE 4.2:   Budget information for Small Australian Research Council Grant—Constructing Toxic Shock Syndrome: Selected Australian Print-based Media Representations of Toxic Shock Syndrome 1979-1995.

Detailed Budget Items	Priority	Amount Requested		
		1996	**1997** ARC Small Grants only	**1998** ARC Small Grants only
Personnel				
Research Assistant Step 1 ($29,554)				
Phase 1 - 0.6x4 months x 29,554	A	**$5912.00**		
Phase 2 - 0.4x5 months x 29,554	A	**$4925.00**		
Phase 3 - 0.2x3 months x 29,554	A	**$1478.00**		

		$12,315.00		
+ 13.2 Oncosts		**$1,625.00**		

		$13,940.00		
Clerical Assistant 20 hours x $15.00	A	**$300.00**		
Maintenance				
Costs associated with locating and obtaining articles	A	**$2,000.00**		
Printing	A	**$200.00**		
General Photocopying (eg of drafts)	A	**$50.00**		

Financial summary

Support requested	Personnel $	Equipment $	Maintenance $	Travel $	Vessel $	Other $	Total $
1996	14,240	2,000	250				16,490.00
1997 (ARC Small Grants)							
1998 (ARC Small Grants)							

The justification, that is, the reason why each budget item requested is essential for the study to proceed, was as follows:

Research Assistant:

The research assistant will be required to locate, and obtain a copy of each article about Toxic Shock Syndrome. They will also (under supervision) enter the descriptive statistics and the articles found pertaining to Toxic Shock Syndrome. This will require them to be employed 0.6 time during Phase 1 (4 months).

During Phase 2 the research assistant will assist the principal researcher's theming of the articles. This will require them to work 0.4 time (for 5 months). They will also collect any remaining articles in the 1st part of this 5 months.

In the final analysis (Phase 3) they will be required to assist in the analysis, drafting and production of the final form of the research report. They will be required at 0.2 time (for 3 months).

Clerical Assistant:

The clerical assistant will be required for the typing of the progressive drafts and the final report of the research.

Search for, location and copying of articles:

Given that the exact number of articles to be photocopied is unknown, a sum of $2,000 has been allowed based on the following indicative costs, worked on an average of 26 articles (one every 2 weeks) per year per publication:

TABLE 4.3: Costing for Magazine and Newspaper Searches from Small Australian Research Council Grant - Constructing Toxic Shock Syndrome: Selected Australian Print-based Media Representations of Toxic Shock Syndrome 1979-1995.

Location	Magazine/Newspaper	Cost (no. years x articles x cost per page)	Total Cost
Mortlock Library	*Women's Weekly* 1984-1995	12x26x50 cents	$156.00
	Cleo 1979-1989	12x26x50 cents	$156.00
Barr Smith Library	*Advertiser* 1979-1995	17x26x13 cents	$58.00
Flinders University	*Women's Weekly* 1979-1983	5x26x14 cents	$18.50
Dolly Magazine	*Dolly* 1979-1995	17x26x50 cents + $150.00 (fee for contents page photocopying)	$371.00
Cleo Magazine	*Cleo* 1990-1994	5x26x50 cents + $50.00 (fee for contents pages photocopying)	$115.00
Marion Library, Sturt Branch	*Cleo* 1995	1x26x50 cents	$13.00
PRESSCOM	*Advertiser* (searches)		$480.00
		SUBTOTAL	**$1,510.20**
Contingency	if significant number of extra articles are found		$489.80
		TOTAL	**$2,000.00**

Maintenance:
The amount allowed for printing will cover the cost of production of the final report.

You should have noticed that the justification of each component of the budget clearly relates to the identified phases and aims of the project. This is very important as otherwise the reason for requesting a certain component of the budget may not be clear. If you are requesting research assistance, it is important to state clearly in detail why you need the assistance and how it pertains to the research plan and aims of the project. Similarly, specific details need to be provided about maintenance and/or photocopying costs. Table 4.3 is quite detailed. From this table, it is clear that the researcher has done his or her "homework" in ascertaining likely and realistic costs associated with the proposed project. Nothing is more off-putting than an unrealistic or unjustified budget!

CONCLUDING COMMENTS

This chapter has been about the craft of proposal writing and how this craft affects the development of research proposals from postmodern and poststructural perspectives. The discussion has focused on a particular research proposal and has used the analysis of the construction of that proposal to illuminate principles involved in the construction of a proposal. In particular, the need for congruence between the aims, the methods and the theoretical orientation of the project has been emphasized.

We have explored the construction of a research proposal, and have mentioned in passing the notion of a research proposal itself as a form of text complete with its own assumptions and understandings about reality. Building on this, the next chapter focuses on the type of data collected in this study and how that data was analyzed, thereby giving valuable insights into the analytic phase of the postmodern and poststructural research endeavour.

FURTHER READING

Brink, P. & Wood, M. (1994). *Basic steps in planning nursing research: From question to proposal* (4th ed.). Boston: Jones & Bartlett Publishers.

> This book provides a step-by-step guide to planning nursing research. Of particular interest is chapter 13 "Writing the Research Proposal", which provides an in-depth discussion of the different aspects of a research proposal.

Hamilton, H. & Gray, G. (1992). *A guide to successful grant applications: Grant application know how*. Melbourne, Australia: Royal College of Nursing, Australia.

> This booklet was produced by the Australian Royal College of Nursing to help inexperienced nursing researchers gain funding for research. As such, it addresses many of the issues discussed in this chapter, including what constitutes a "good" proposal, choosing an appropriate funding agency, answering the different parts of a grant application successfully, and demonstrating effective management and use of grant monies.

Lupton, D. (1994a). Analysing news coverage. In S. Chapman & D. Lupton (Eds.), *The fight for public health: Principles and practice of media advocacy*. London: BMJ.

> This chapter contextualizes news media coverage of public health issues, highlighting the social pressures that act to construct newsworthy stories. Lupton introduces the principles of discourse analysis, focusing on different parts of a print media article. She suggests means by which the researcher can look beyond the surface content to the subtextual themes evident in the report and to the social context in which the article is produced.

Chapter 5

Speaking Practically, Part 2:
"Doing" Research Informed by Postmodern and Poststructural Approaches

INTRODUCTION

Each research perspective has its own approach to the management and the subsequent analysis of material collected in a research project. For example, if an essentially statistically-based survey was being conducted, then the rules of statistics would be used to analyze the numerical data collected, thereby giving one view of the reality being studied. Similarly if one were to employ a grounded theory research approach, then Glaser and Strauss (1967), Glaser (1978), Glaser (1992) and Strauss and Corbin (1990) provide some clear principles about the management and analysis of the collected material.

It is a little more difficult to point to a set of rules or guidelines for the management and analysis of information collected in postmodern and poststructural research. Such difficulty arises, at least in part, from a point made earlier in this book: that is, there is not just one approach or method to research using postmodern or poststructural perspectives. Indeed, as Rosenau (1992) points out, "post-modernists are not inclined to use the word method, though they sometimes discuss "strategies" or "struggles" around truth and knowledge in terms that approximate methodology" (p. 116).

What Rosenau highlights about method in postmodern studies also applies to the analysis of the material collected in these studies. Thus, rather than discussing analytical techniques or procedures applicable to all postmodern or poststructural research, this chapter explores struggles and strategies in the analysis of the material collected in a specific study to highlight how one might go about analyzing this data. However, it is important to note that the result of exploring such struggles and strategies is neither definitive answers nor portrayals of "reality". This is because:

> post-modern social science presumes methods that multiply paradox, inventing ever more elaborate repertoires of questions, each of which encourages an infinity of answers, rather than methods that settle on solutions. (Rosenau 1992, p. 117).

Discussion or analytical endeavour from a postmodern or poststructural frame is explicit about the ability of any research to capture only partial realities and partial understandings. Any research approach takes a particular position from which to view and/or describe the reality in question.

With this in mind, we will now consider what the material collected in the study outlined in Chapter 4 "looked like" and what strategies and struggles were employed in its analysis. We will explore each phase of the study to try to get a "feel" for the way in which the study and the subsequent analyses were conducted. In particular, we will explore the discursive focus of the analysis that occurred in Phase 3 of the study. The rationale for taking such an approach is similar to that given by Parker (1992) for developing an understanding of discourse analysis:

> Perhaps the best way to get a feel for forms of discourse [strategies and struggles] is to look at how analysts actually deal with texts [empirical materials collected in studies]. (Parker 1992, p. 127)

COLLECTING AND ANALYZING THE MATERIAL: PHASE 1 OF THE STUDY

You will remember that Phase 1 of this study (see Chapter 4, "Research plan, methods and techniques") was concerned with outlining the extent, range, location, timing and type of reporting of issues in particular media concerning toxic shock syndrome (TSS). Thirteen categories for the analysis were given:

1 Headline
2 Topic
3 Visual material
4 Sources quoted
5 Whether it is primarily theoretical or practical
6 Tone—positive or negative?
7 Position in paper/magazine
8 Relationship (if any) to other news articles at the time
9 Type of print media it appears in
10 Type of audience article is pitched at
11 Day of week
12 Month of year
13 Year

The identification of the categories to be used was initially drawn from other research (e.g. Lupton (1994a)—categories 1,2,3,4; Chrisler and Levy (1990)—categories 5,6.

The first step in the analysis was to actually locate the articles! In all, 68 articles were found: 34 from *The Advertiser,* 16 from *Dolly,* 12 from *Cleo* and 6 from *The Australian Women's Weekly* (see Table 1 in appendix B). However, before it was possible to begin analyzing each article in terms of the listed categories, it was necessary to state clearly what understanding or definition of each category was being used. For example, with respect to the category, headline, the following research notes were made:

Headlines
1. Summarize the main topic of the story
2. Are designed to capture readers' attention through considered choice of language and through presenting the crux of story in as few words as possible.
3. Signify to the reader how to "define" the situation or events reported.
4. Can be analyzed in terms of:

   - tone e.g. horror, shock, the bizarre, informative, neutral
   - conspicuousness—headline size in relation to surrounding articles
     - headline in bold writing
     - style of writing (e.g. normal or italicized)
   - prominence—position of articles on page
   - content

Having established the broad categories for analysis, we developed codes for each category. Some of these codes were modified from previous research. For example, Gabe, Gustaffson and Bury's (1991) five-part categorization of print media provided the initial codes for the category types of print media. Alternatively codes emerged from the data obtained from the identification of commonly occurring themes (for example, the codes pertaining to the tone of headlines). The definition of each code was given so that it was clear what understandings were informing the research. Once a clear framework of categories and their related codes had been established, it was possible to code each article and use descriptive statistics to show the extent, range, location, timing and type of reporting of issues concerning TSS in the media.

For example, from the notes developed about the category of headline, a coding system for analysis of the articles in terms of headline characteristics was developed and was constantly refined as articles were read and coded. The final coding system is outlined as follows.

Codes For The Category "Headline"

1. Number of article (identification purposes)
2. Tone
   1 Shock
   2 Discreditory
   3 Neutral
   4 Reassuring
   5 Bizarre
   6 Poignant
   7 Informative
   8 Warning
   9 Speculative
   10 Legal
   11 No headline
3. Conspicuousness: Headline size in relation to surrounding articles
   1 Small
   2 Medium
   3 Large
   4 Extra large
   5 No headline
4. Conspicuousness: Headline in bold writing
   1 Yes
   2 No
   3 No headline
5. Conspicuousness: Style of writing
   1 Normal
   2 Italicized
   3 In negative
   4 Varying styles/fonts
   5 No headline
6. Prominence: Position of article on the page
   1 Entire page
   2 Top left
   3 Top central
   4 Top right
   5 Left central
   6 Central
   7 Right central
   8 Bottom left
   9 Bottom central
   10 Bottom right
7. Content of headline
   1 TSS as a killer disease of young women
   2 TSS as associated with tampon use
   3 TSS as caused by tampon use
   4 TSS as unrelated to tampon use

5   TSS as a problem of tampon production
6   TSS as an unknown quantity
7   TSS as a known quantity/latest information
8   TSS as a disease of tampon hygiene
9   TSS as a disease that the individual can prevent
10 Tampons are safe
11 Tampons are dangerous
12 TSS and Peta-Ann Devine
13 TSS as a serious condition
14 TSS as questionable
15 Neutral
16 Other

As stated previously, it was important that what was meant or understood by each code was clearly stated. Thus, for example, the following definitions were developed for the codes under the "tone" section of the analysis of the headline.

Shock: Headlines designed to grab attention through causing surprise or fear including those playing on the word "shock"; for example, "'Scary' new disease kills women" (Wilson 1980, p.1).

Discreditory: A headline that casts doubt on the accuracy, authority or reputation of something or someone. For example, headlines that cast doubt on specific cases of TSS, or the cause of TSS, such as, "Tampons 'not linked' to toxic shock" (Rice 1989, p.8).

Neutral: Headlines that don't take sides, such as headlines that signify content and are usually only one- or two-word headlines, for example, "Tampons" (Tampons 1985, p.154).

Reassuring: Headlines designed to restore confidence in a particular brand of tampons or a companys such as Johnson & Johnson. One example of such a headline is "Carefree tampons cleared of blame" (Hailstone 1981, p.9).

Bizarre: Headlines which involve sensational content, or incongruities, or bringing together sensational elements such as "Toxic shock in transsexual" (King 1983, p.141).

Poignant: Headlines designed to play on feelings and evoke an emotional reaction, such as personalized accounts of the effects of TSS: for example, "A schoolgirl's last moment's" ("A schoolgirl" 1995, p. 4).

Informative: Headlines that convey facts without emotional content, headlines giving information or headlines indicating that the article will give information: for example, "Toxic shock report" (Brooks 1995, pp. 54-6).

Warning: Headlines that give notice of a potential danger or indicate that the article will do so: for example, "Tampon warning" ("Tampon warning" 1980, p. 2).

Speculative: Headlines that indicate that information and facts about TSS and/or tampons are questionable, sometimes suggesting the need for further inquiry into TSS or tampons: for example, "T.S.S.: Mystery disease linked with tampons" ("T.S.S.: Mystery" 1981, p. 118).

Legal: Headlines that refer to legal processes or alternately use legal language such as "Woman sues tampon maker" ("Woman sues tampon maker" *1989*, p. 5).

Once these codes had been established it was possible to code each article in terms of the headline category. For example, consider the following article:

'Scary' new disease kills women

Doctors in the US are being altered to a new disease that hits mostly young women and can cause death within a few days.

It is called 'toxic-shock syndrome' and 55 cases have been reported in the US since October.

The Federal Centre for Disease Control said 52 of those victims were women and seven of them had died.

Spokeswoman Dr. Kathryn Shands described the disease as 'scary'.

Most people, she said, didn't seek medical attention quickly enough because the initial symptoms were similar to those of a minor virus infection.

Most victims had been women who had started a menstrual period no more than five days before falling ill.

They then developed a fever, diarrhoea and vomiting, sometimes accompanied by headaches, sore throat and aching muscles.

Within two days, the victims went into shock. Their blood pressure fell, often producing kidney failure and disorientation.

At the same time, they developed a patchy red rash, sometimes caused the skin to peel.

'Most people don't seek care until they get dizziness or collapse from shock,' Dr. Shands said.

Thirteen patients had had the disease more than once.

'If it recurs, it is likely to return during a menstrual period but not necessarily the next month,' Dr. Shands said.

'No one knows why almost all of the victims are women.'

The Wisconsin State Health Department became aware of the disease in December and sent a letter all Wisconsin doctors describing it.

Experts have since analysed specimens from the blood, urine, skin and mouths of toxic-shock patients in search of its cause.

'They suspect that it may be produced by a toxin – or poison – from a bacterium,' Dr. Shands said.

'We hope that doctors across the United States will now begin to recognise the disease and report other cases.'

The coding that was used for this article with respect to its headline was:

– Tone—shock
– Conspicuousness: headline size in relation to surrounding articles—medium
– Conspicuousness: headline in bold—no
– Conspicuousness: style of writing—normal
– Prominence: position of article on the page—central
– Content of headline—TSS as a killer disease of young women.

The article was then analyzed in terms of the other categories specified in the research proposal, and the codes that had been developed for those categories.

It is not possible in the space of one chapter to analyze each category and its associated codes in detail. However, if you examine Appendix B closely you will get an idea of the categories and codes that were used. The tables there represent the descriptive statistics about the articles developed in Phase 1 of this analysis. Hopefully, the detailed discussion of the category "headline" and the way in which codes were developed about this category will give valuable insights into how such coding can occur.

PHASE 2: QUALITATIVE THEMATIC ANALYSIS: DEVELOPING A CHRONOLOGY OF TOPICS

In this phase of the study, the 68 articles were analyzed qualitatively in terms of the themes that were present in the reporting about TSS. Following Lupton (1994c), a chronology of the reporting about TSS in these four media sources was developed.

TABLE 5.2 Chronology of the Topics Appearing in Articles in *The Advertiser*, *The Australian Women's Weekly, Dolly and Cleo* About Toxic Shock Syndrome, 1979-95.
Reprinted with the permission of Sage Publications Ltd. From Cheek, J. "(Con)textualizing Toxic Shock Syndrome: Selected Media Representations of the Emergence of a Health Phenomenon 1979-1995", Sage publIcations Pty Ltd., 1997.

Jan.-June 1980	Emergence of TSS as a women's disease of unknown origin /signs and symptoms (*The Advertiser*)
July-Dec. 1980	TSS as a disease arising from Rely Tampons (*The Advertiser*) New Zealand women advised against the use of tampons after a local TSS death (*The Advertiser*)
	continued

Jan.-June 1981	First reported case of TSS in Australia /links with carefree tampons (*The Advertiser*)
	Withdrawal of Carefree tampons produced in New Zealand after a second reported case of TSS (*The Advertiser*)
	Carefree tampons found to be uncontaminated /information about preventative hygiene measures (*The Advertiser*)
	TSS death in the United States (*The Advertiser*)
	Australian TSS victim discharged/ no evidence of staphylococcus aureus in Carefree tampons (*The Advertiser*)
	TSS as a staphylococcus aureus infection predominantly associated with women using tampons/ speculation about possible causes for this link (*The Australian Women's Weekly*)
	TSS as a staphylococcus aureus disease affecting both sexes, but predominantly seen in menstruating women (*The Australian Women's Weekly*)
	General information about TSS as a new disease linked with tampon use/speculation on its causes/ preventative hygiene measures (*Cleo*)
July-Dec. 1981	Article presenting the pros and cons of tampon use /TSS related to problems with tampon production (*Dolly*)
	General information about TSS/ downplays the threat of TSS in Australia /TSS presented as caused by abrasions to the vaginal wall (*Dolly*)
Jan.-June 1982	Legal proceedings against Gamble and Proctor (makers of Rely tampons) due to a TSS death in the United States. (*The Advertiser*)
	Court orders Gamble and Proctor to pay out the TSS victim. (*The Advertiser*)
	General information about TSS/presented as a disease of men as well/ calls for volunteers for further research (*The Advertiser*)
	Update on means of infection in TSS /TSS as transmitted on women's hands from skin infections (*The Australian Women's Weekly*)
July-Dec. 1982	TSS as a disease of both sexes acquired after surgery /TSS as a staphylococcal infection (*Cleo*)
Jan.-June 1983	TSS as an auto immune condition furthered by the mechanics of tampon use (trapping of air in vagina) (*The Advertiser*)
	TSS as a disease of both sexes caused by staphylococcus aureus (*The Australian Women's Weekly*)
	TSS in a male transsexual after chemical face peel/ TSS as a staphylococcal infection(*Cleo*)

continued

July-Dec. 1983	General information about safe tampon use/Downplays the threat of TSS in Australia (*Dolly*)
	General information about menstruation and tampon use/ TSS as a rare disease (Cleo)
	Retention of an old tampon and the possibility of TSS (*Cleo*)
Jan.-June 1984	Links TSS to mechanics of tampon insertion (*The Advertiser*)
July-Dec. 1984	
Jan.-June 1985	General information about TSS/presented as a rare disease/ prevention of TSS through regularly changing tampons (*Dolly*)
	TSS as a disease caused by germs "produced in tampons"/ Downplays current danger (*Dolly*)
	TSS presented as a rare disease/preventative hygiene measures (*Cleo* as sponsored by Johnson & Johnson Pty Ltd)
	General menstrual information/ TSS as a disease related to tampon retention (*Cleo* as sponsored by Johnson & Johnson Pty Ltd)
	TSS as related to Rely tampons and caused by the 'toxin produced by a particular species of germ called staph' (*Cleo* as sponsored by Johnson & Johnson Pty Ltd)
July-Dec. 1985	TSS from tampon retention/preventative hygiene measures (Dolly)
Jan.-June 1986	The establishment of voluntary standards for tampon production and packaging (*The Advertiser*)
	TSS presented as a disease related to American tampons and caused by a 'toxin produced by a bacterium....called staph. aureus' (*Cleo* as sponsored by Johnson & Johnson Pty Ltd)
June-Dec. 1986	
Jan.-June 1987	Preventative hygiene measures/ 'TSS... isn't caused by tampons' (but by) 'golden staph. which can grow on a neglected tampon' (*Cleo* as sponsored by Johnson & Johnson)
July-Dec. 1987	
Jan.-June 1988	
July-Dec. 1988	
Jan.-June 1989	14-year-old. British girl dies after retaining a tampon for 48 hours (*The Advertiser*)
July-Dec. 1989	Australian victim of TSS (Janette Thompson) sues Johnson & Johnson (*The Advertiser*)
	Dismissal of the Jury in case against Johnson & Johnson due to comments made on the radio about the trial (*The Advertiser*)
	Side effects of TSS as presented to the court in the trial against Johnson & Johnson. (*The Advertiser*)
	Legal defence in case against Johnson & Johnson /"No statistical link between Toxic shock Syndrome and the use of tampons" (*The Advertiser*) Johnson & Johnson cleared of claims of negligence (*The Advertiser*) *continued*

	Statement by Johnson & Johnson about safe production methods of tampons and nappies (*The Australian Women's Weekly*)
	Answers concerns about bleaches and dyes in tampons /TSS as a disease that has been controlled through the removal of dangerous tampons from the market (*Dolly*)
Jan.-June 1990	Statistical reduction in TSS linked to changes in tampon production (*The Advertiser*)
July-Dec. 1990	
Jan.-June 1991	
July-Dec 1991	Information about pros and cons of tampon use/ Relates TSS to the retention of tampons (*The Australian Women's Weekly*)
Jan.-June 1992	
July-Dec. 1992	Signs and symptoms of TSS/ TSS related to tampon retention/ self-help advice (*Dolly*)
Jan.-June 1993	
July-Dec. 1993	Information about the retention of tampons and TSS (*Cleo*)
Jan.-June 1994	Safety of tampon use-preventative hygiene measures/ TSS as a disease associated with the use of super absorbent tampons (*Dolly*) TSS as a tampon-related bacterial infection that can be treated medically/ preventative hygiene measures (*Dolly*)
July-Dec. 1994	Article about the pros and cons of different forms of sanitary protection /TSS as a bacterial disease associated with super absorbent tampons(*Dolly*) TSS as a bacterial infection caused by tampons /preventative hygiene measures/ information about insertion of tampons (*Dolly*) General information about TSS/ TSS as a result of tampon retention leading to an appropriate culture for the 'germs' that cause TSS (*Cleo*)
Jan.-June 1995	General information on TSS after the death of Peta-Ann Devine /review of the standards of tampon production (*The Advertiser*) Detection of a bacterial infection in some blood supplies (constructed as Toxic Shock) (*The Advertiser*) Moves to introduce compulsory health warnings on tampon packages (*The Advertiser*) Account of Peta-Ann Devine's death from TSS/ information about standards for tampon production (*The Advertiser*) General medical information about TSS from a warning on American tampon packages (*The Advertiser*) Establishment of the TSS information service (*The Advertiser*) Establishment of a free TSS hotline (*The Advertiser*) Peta-Ann Devine's father calls for standards for tampon production (*The Advertiser*) *continued*

	Proceedings of the first inquest into Peta-Ann Devine's death (*The Advertiser*)
	Inquest finds that Peta-Ann Devine's death was not caused by TSS (*The* Advertiser)
	Application lodged to reopen inquest into Peta-Ann Devine's death (*The Advertiser*)
	Tampon packets to carry health warning (*The Advertiser*)
	General article about menstrual cycle/TSS as a rare bacterial infection that releases toxins/ presentative hygiene measures (*Dolly*)
July-Dec. 1995	New inquest into Peta-Ann Devine's death scheduled (*Advertiser*)
	Report of coroner's finding in Peta-Ann Devine inquest /TSS is not responsible (*Dolly*)
	TSS as a staphylococcal infection that can be fatal due to a lack of antibodies /two personalised accounts of TSS (*Dolly*)
	Preventative hygiene measures /clinical testing for antibodies (*Dolly*)

At this stage, the analysis was still in the realm of the descriptive rather than the discursive. The chronology presents the themes pertaining to the content of the reporting about TSS. An interesting aspect to emerge from the chronology about the content of the reporting of TSS concerned shifts in emphasis in the reporting. TSS went from being constructed largely as a problem of individual women and their menstrual hygiene to being presented as a problem of tampon production.

PHASE 3: ANALYZING THE REPORTING ABOUT TOXIC SHOCK SYNDROME DISCURSIVELY

Phases 1 and 2 of the study provided a description of what was reported about TSS as well as detail about how it was reported both in terms of its actual physical presentation in the media and the angle or slant used to construct the discussion. The final phase (Phase 3) of the study moved the analysis from the descriptive to the discursive. The emphasis in this phase was on the way TSS has been represented discursively in the media and on what such representation exposes about assumptions and understandings of TSS, health and illness.

It is important to emphasize yet again that there is not just one method or set of guidelines that can be posited and then followed with respect to discourse analysis. You may remember Parker's (1992) assertion quoted in Chapter 3 that discourse analysis "is not, or should not be, a 'method' to be wheeled on and applied to any and every topic" (p. 122). Accordingly, the analysis in Phase 3 of this study used a series of strategies and struggles to explore the articles discursively. The guiding question was: "What discourses frame these texts and in turn are framed by such texts?". Thus, the articles were explored as much in terms of the unstated and unspoken assumptions framing them as in terms of those that were stated. Parker's questions "Why was this said, and not that? Why these words, and where do the connotations of the words fit with different ways of talking about the world?" (p. 4) provided a useful starting point.

Each article was read and Parker's questions were asked. For example, consider the article "'Scary' new disease kills women" reproduced in Figure 5.1 (Wilson 1980, p. 1). It appeared on the front page of *The Advertiser*—the first time the newspaper had reported TSS.

Examples of questions that can be asked about the way this article has been framed include:

–   Why was the word "scary" used and not another word?

–   What connotations does the word "scary" have?

–   TSS is referred to a "new disease". Where does this locate TSS and how will such a location affect the way TSS is viewed by women, health professionals and others?

–   Women with TSS are referred to as "victims". What is the effect of this word? How does it locate or situate women with respect to TSS?

–   Who speaks authoritatively about TSS and what enables them to be able to do so?

–   Who or what is absent from such a report? For example, notice the invisibility of tampons from the construction of understandings of TSS at this point in time.

It is apparent from this article that TSS is being framed by, and located within, scientific/medical discourse. TSS is described in terms of its physiological symptoms and incidence rate. Thus it is those whose expertise draws on scientific/medical frames who are able to speak with authority about both what TSS is and how it might be managed. The unstated assumption is that it is a biological syndrome and that science will provide the solution. The "disease" TSS officially exists now, as it has been formally recognized by the Federal Centre for Disease Control. Finally, it is interesting to note that there is the first hint of what will become a prominent frame in subsequent articles, namely that "victims" of TSS acted in some way to bring about the onset of the syndrome: "most people...didn't seek medical attention quickly enough" (Wilson 1980, p.1).

Each article located about TSS was explored by asking questions about the way it was framed so that both the understandings implicit in the way TSS was reported and the understandings constructed about TSS by such representation would be uncovered and exposed.

What, then, did the analysis uncover? What discursive frames influenced the way TSS was represented in the media? What was the effect of these frames? The rest of the discussion about this phase of the study, and in particular, the answers to these questions, is adapted from an article of mine published in *Health: An Interdisciplinary Journal for the Social Study of Health, Illness and Medicine.* (From Cheek, J., (Con)textualizing Toxic Shock Syndrome: Selected media representations of the emergence of a health phenomenon 1979-1995, pp 188-189 & 190-200. Copyright 1997 by Sage Publications 1997. Adapted with permission.)

I begin the discussion by reviewing the concept of discourse and then move on to discuss the major discursive frames implicit within the reporting that is done about TSS. Finally, I trouble the concept of a "passive" reader of texts about TSS, arguing that there is a need for further study to investigate how readers of these articles actually understand and respond to the texts.

REPORT ON THE FINDINGS OF PHASE 3 ANALYSIS

Discourses refer to ways of thinking and talking about reality. They are "practices that systematically form the objects of which they speak" (Foucault 1974, p. 49): they constitute them and in the practice of so doing conceal their own intention. "A discourse provides a set of possible statements about a given area, and organises and gives structure to the manner in which a particular topic, object, process is to be talked about" (Kress 1985, p.7). As Parker (1992) puts it, "discourses do not simply describe the social world, but categorise it, they bring phenomena into sight ... Discourses provide frameworks for debating the value of one way of talking about reality over other ways" (pp. 4-5). Implicit within Parker's statement is the notion that there are different possibilities for talking about reality at any point in time. However, not all ways of talking and thinking about a particular aspect of reality, for example TSS, may be afforded equal value. Dominant discursive frameworks may actually have the effect of limiting, or even excluding, other possibilities for thinking about the reality in question. Hence "discourse is not simply that which translates struggles or systems of domination, but is the thing for which, and by which, there is struggle, discourse is the power which is to be seized" (Foucault 1984, p. 110).

Discourses, therefore, enable what may be said or written about a particular object or health issue, for example TSS, at a particular time, but in so doing, limit the possibility of alternate views being presented. As Morley (1992) puts it: "While the message is not an object with one real meaning, there are within it signifying mechanisms which promote certain meanings, even one privileged meaning, and suppress others" (p. 21). The way in which TSS is represented in the media involves the creation of certain viewing positions for the readers of articles. The articles collected from the newspaper and popular magazines promote certain understandings of TSS and suppress others. The power of dominant discourses to frame public understandings of issues, including those pertaining to health, has been illustrated by Workman (1996) in his incisive analysis of the way in which dominant discourse of fiscal debt reported incessantly in the media "domesticates or colonizes understanding(s)" (p. 31); "assigns seriousness and establishes concern" (p.30) and ultimately "disciplines the dialogue" (p.31) that is possible about monetary policy in Canada.

Workman concludes:

> The discourse of fiscal crisis, in summary, assigns seriousness, fixes truth, establishes the margins of debate, disciplines participants, domesticates understanding, confirms comprehension, mediates information and routinizes discussion. (p. 31)

What then are the discourses that shape the representation of, and understandings about, TSS and ultimately discipline the dialogue about it? How is seriousness assigned, truth fixed, understandings domesticated and discussion routinized about this relatively recent health phenomena? Three major discursive frameworks were identified as shaping the writing and representation in the articles found about TSS: the discourse of concealment, scientific/medical discourse and discourses about individual responsibility for health. This is not to say there are not others, but that in this particular study these were the major discursive frames to emerge. Each of these discourses and the understandings and representations of TSS they convey is now explored in more detail.

Mentioning the Unmentionable—Discourses of Concealment

Discourses surrounding TSS are particularly problematic as TSS touches on such taboo areas as menstruation and sanitary products (Delaney, Lupton & Toth 1988). Ms. Thompson is reported as stating during her court proceedings against Johnson & Johnson she "feel[s] very embarrassed ... it is something so personal" ("Woman sues tampon maker" 1989, p.5). Discussions about TSS, related as they inevitably are to menstruation and tampon use, contravene a powerful social discourse which Laws (1990) refers to as menstrual etiquette—"the intricate social rules that people in society attach to it" (p. 43).

Menstrual etiquette is a powerful subtextual frame in the reporting of TSS which determines how the menses are to be "dealt" with and above all "requires that no-one should know, unless she chooses to tell" (Ginsburg 1996, p. 370). Discussions about TSS and its link to tampon use inevitably make visible an otherwise concealed phenomenon. By going to court and giving public evidence about her use of tampons Ms. Thompson contravened the unwritten and unspoken social rules of menstrual etiquette. Thus it is no surprise that Ms. Thompson should report feelings of embarrassment and discomfort at exposing hitherto invisible and unspoken details of menstruation and tampon use. She had not behaved in the "normal" way of concealing such details in line with what have become commonsense and taken-for-granted understandings of how to behave with respect to menstruation. Menstrual etiquette demands that discussion and details of menstruation be purposefully absent. Such purposeful absences and "women's efforts to make sense of their absences ... inform our ideology of femininity, and ultimately corroborate dominant society's views about the status of women" (Ginsburg 1996, p. 367).

A bodily function affecting over half the population at some stage of their life has thus been constructed in the discourse of its private, personal and fundamentally invisible nature. Such a discourse creates the need and desire for "sanitary protection" that is discreet—for example with no bulges—thereby enabling women to keep their secret safe (Delaney et al. 1988). These "feminine hygiene" products are designed to "conceal and/or eliminate all indicators of menstrual status and thereby provide an antidote to the experience of tainted femininity" (Block Coutts & Berg 1993, p.186). These products are packaged in such a way as to conceal what they are and what they are to be used for—"the very design of menstrual products encourages their discretionary handling" (Ginsburg 1996, p. 367). Such "protection" in the form of pads and tampons is part of the discourse of concealment framing menstrual etiquette and is rarely to be discussed.

Ginsburg (1996) relates the desire to conceal both the fact of menstruation itself and the products used to assist in achieving such invisibility, to the participation of women in a male-centred world, arguing that "compliance with menstrual etiquette recalls to women their status as objects, diverts their attention, and compels them to participate in the male gaze" (1996, p. 365). Operating as if under the scrutiny of an ever-present male, women are expected to "buy, store and use them [sanitary products] without men noticing" (Laws 1990, p. 45). One can never be sure who is watching, when. There is an ever-present panoptic gaze (Foucault 1977). Concealment is paramount and women monitor and police their behaviour in order to comply with this powerful discursive frame. Put another way, in terms of the desire to conceal the fact of menstruation:

> in contemporary patriarchal culture, a panoptical male connoisseur resides within the consciousness of most women: they stand perpetually before his gaze and under his judgment. Woman lives her body as seen by another, by an anonymous patriarchal Other (Bartky 1988, p.72).

Thus, Delaney et al. (1988,), note that women's function with respect to feminine hygiene is to "deodorize, sanitize and remove the evidence" (p. 107). Yet the paradox is that, "as hidden as menstrual products are, they are also ever-present" (Ginsburg 1996, p. 366). Every 28 days or so, many women will use and handle these hidden objects. The discourse of concealment, framed by the unmentionable nature of menstruation and menstrual products, creates a tension in the reporting of TSS, a syndrome so clearly linked to such "unmentionables".. What had previously been carefully relegated to the margins suddenly assumes centre frame—but only in connection with a potentially lethal syndrome, often reported in a sensational manner by the press.

The Scientific/Medical Frame

The impact of scientific/medical discourse both in defining TSS itself and assigning seriousness in terms of risk, was apparent throughout the entire period in which TSS was reported in the media. The first reports of TSS in *The Advertiser* reflect a sceptical attitude on the part of some doctors to reports of TSS in the United States. Indeed, the second article to appear in *The Advertiser* (Kennedy 1980) quotes a medical professor from the Queen Elizabeth Hospital as stating that "from the medical point of view there should not be any disease from such a trivial matter" (p. 29)! This statement reveals the power of medical discourse—that is medical ways of thinking and talking about aspects of reality—to define what diseases are and even if diseases exist, despite the obvious lack of knowledge about TSS at this time by the doctors involved. As Backhouse (1996) points out:

> the social and subjective nature of medical knowledge is very strongly demonstrated by the paradox that while medicine is largely legitimated through its scientific rigour and effectiveness, it is often in practice afforded very high levels of credibility and acceptance *before* its efficacy has been scientifically established (1996, p.188, emphasis in original).

Indeed the same article in *The Advertiser* reports a comment from another doctor as "I'm inclined to think it's another American beat-up to scare the nation's females" (p. 29). The use of the word "trivial", presumably in reference to the use of tampons during menstruation, and the patronizing tone of the statement "to scare the nation's females' reflect a certain view of women's health and women themselves. Perhaps this is why, 15 years on, *The Advertiser,* in reporting the findings of a Therapeutic Goods Administration report into standards of tampon production, notes that the incidence of TSS is still unknown and that the public should be made aware of the illness (Kerr 1995a, p.33).

From the outset then, scientific/medical discourse defined firstly whether TSS existed, and then when research demonstrated that TSS did indeed exist, what could or could not be identified as TSS. The power of the scientific/medical frame to determine not only the definition of the disease but what counted in the determination of that definition was clearly evident from the reporting of the first inquest in 1995 into Peta-Ann Devine's death, where debate centred around whether Peta-Ann did, or did not, die from TSS. When writing about the debate in the courts about whether Peta-Ann Devine had died from TSS, Garland (who is Chair of a Toxic Shock Syndrome panel backed by tampon manufacturers) and Peel (1995) were able to draw on medical/scientific discursive frames to assert:

> the syndrome of toxic shock is based on a constellation of strict diagnostic criteria, and unless the girl's signs and symptoms complied with these TSS cannot be diagnosed. Unfortunately this consideration did not stop sections of the Australian media attributing the girl's death to TSS (Garland and Peel 1995, p.8).

Thus, when TSS was established as a "legitimate" disease by those who could claim expert knowledge (Freidson 1970), it was defined according to medical/scientific discourse. TSS became a set of symptoms, a category of diagnosis, which had the effect of both establishing the margins of debate and routinizing discussion about TSS. Put another way, knowledge about TSS had become seemingly objective—that is stabilized (Guillemin 1996). The "norm" had been established in terms of the medical definition of TSS, and that which did not fit the norm could be dismissed or relegated to "other". Clarke (1991) argues that such "medical definitions...have surpassed religious, and in some instances, legal definitions in their power to direct and provide meaning for human social life" (p. 288). It is thus interesting to note that in the legal judgment handed down in the *Thompson vs Johnson & Johnson* case, scientific/ medical discourse was used to define and frame requisite standards of care of manufacturers to their consumers. As Reid (1991) reports "in ascertaining the requisite standard of care the trial Judge's reasoning emphasized the importance of analysing events in terms of the then current state of scientific knowledge" (p. 182).

However, although such "strict diagnostic criteria" and the "current state of scientific knowledge" may seem objective and factual, Garrett (1994) highlights that they may, in fact, not be. Garrett points out that the basic case definition of TSS developed by the Center for Disease Control (CDC) in the United States was severely criticized for focusing on acute cases only. Thus:

> Among the first 100 cases reported to CDC, the agency selected 43 that met the stringent definition of TSS. That meant 57 cases went unexplored—at least some of which might have proven to be milder manifestations of staph infection. As publicity increased, so did the number of ostensible TSS cases that fell outside of the CDC definition (Garrett 1994, pp. 396-7).

Such criticism of the methodology employed to define TSS challenges notions of objective, value-free scientific/medical frames. What counts, and even more importantly what does not count, in such frames is often far from objective. Thus as Collyer (1996) asserts:

> The reputation of the researchers and public credibility of the sponsoring company have a significant impact on the number of tests completed, the selection of the subjects and trial protocols and the results of the trials. This social shaping of the process can become apparent when the results of the trial are publicly contested (p. 11).

Hence, "neither the experience of disease...nor the scientific facts which explain it have an objective existence outside the social process through which they were created" (Ripper 1991, p. 429).

The power of scientific/medical discourse to define the "truth" about TSS was evident from the way it was reported in popular magazines. Most references to TSS were in the form of health columns or health related replies to readers' questions. In *The Australian Women's Weekly* these were referred to as "Medi-facts". In *Dolly* they were in the section known as "Dolly Doctor". Inevitably responses given were framed as authoritative and factual. Yet an analysis of the articles highlights that even seemingly objective, factual, scientific knowledge can be questionable. For example, in October 1985 a *Dolly* reader asked "Is it safe to go to sleep with a tampon inserted?" ("Tampons" 1985, p.154). The answer given was "Yes—it's quite Okay" (p. 154). Compare this to the advice given in *Dolly* in July 1995: "Never sleep with a tampon in place, use sanitary pads" (Brooks 1995, p. 56). Whilst it is quite understandable that knowledge about health phenomena changes over time there is no recognition of this in these replies. Purported medical-based knowledge in these magazines is inevitably framed as authoritative and definitive, as timeless truths. The type of reporting in "Dolly Doctor" and *The Australian Women's Weekly's* "Medi-facts" encourages such a view.

The scientific/medical frame is central in creating perceptions of risk with respect to TSS. As Stallings (1990) points out:

> the reality of risk for most of us exists mainly in images created by others. These images "key note" our collective attempt to make sense out of the world, including its risks, by helping to structure the lines along which initial discussions proceed. (p. 81)

In July 1991, *The Australian Women's Weekly's* "Healthwise" column written by Dr. Frances Mackenzie reports: "The risk of toxic shock being associated with tampons made in Australia is very low—I haven't heard of a case for several years" (1991, p. 117). Similarly, "Dolly Doctor" authoritatively reports in May 1985 that "risks today are minimal and the disease has virtually vanished" ("Could you please explain?" 1985, p. 137). *Cleo* declares in March 1986 in a Cleo/Johnson and Johnson promotion, "TSS is not really an issue in Australia anymore, but the TSS scare led us to be even more careful regarding basic rules of cleanliness when it comes to using tampons" ("I was wondering" 1986, p. 11).

Indeed in August 1994 (just prior to Peta-Ann Devine's death in November 1994) an article in *Dolly* declared: "While some women died many years ago of Toxic Shock Syndrome (TSS)—a disease that was sometimes associated with using super tampons—the risk of getting the disease now is incredibly tiny" (Brooks 1994, p. 105). Since TSS was only named as such in 1979, presumably we can assume that for a teenage audience, 15 years is "many years ago"! This aside, given the "incredibly tiny" risk of TSS espoused by *Dolly* in August 1994, it is interesting to find that an article published in *Dolly* in July 1995 (just after Peta-Ann Devine's death and the first coronial inquest into her death) declared TSS to be something "every girl should know about" (Brooks 1995, p. 54) and a "dangerous condition" (p. 54). It is clear from the few examples given that the risk of TSS is very much a changing phenomenon and that "media attention ... heightens concern, regardless of the degree of risk. Drama, symbolism and identifiable victims, particularly children or celebrities, make the risk more memorable...controversy ensures greater coverage" (Russell 1993, p. 194).

The involvement of the tampon manufacturers in sponsoring information drawing on medical/scientific frames, such as the joint promotion with Johnson & Johnson in *Cleo* 1986 referred to previously, highlights the interconnectedness between the development and dissemination of medical/scientific knowledge and the industries supporting that development. As Collyer (1996), points out, there is a "complex relationship between economic interests and innovation" (p. 17). After all, *Cleo* ("TSS: mystery disease" 1981, p. 118) reports that tampons are an $18 million business. However, all too often, the effects of such a complex relationship in terms of what knowledge is developed, when and by whom, is ignored. It is important to recognize that "the social construction of medical knowledge can be explained as a process of social, political and economic negotiation" (Short 1996, v).

All of this is not to discount the importance of scientific/medical knowledge. Rather, it is to question such knowledge as constituting the definitive and only view of health issues such as TSS. Further, the scientific/medical frame itself, is not a unitary one—within it there are interest and factional groups. As Garrett (1994) somewhat cynically reports:

> The race was on to solve the Toxic Shock mystery and from the outset the investigation was fraught with scientific back stabbing, rivalries, name calling and controversy...there would be little free information for public digestion (p.396).

Discourses about Individual Responsibility for Health

A third powerful discursive frame shaping the reporting of TSS is that of individual responsibility for one's health. This discourse draws on "common assumptions about the role and nature of the individual within contemporary capitalist society in the West" (Workman 1996, p. 71). An emphasis in both the newspaper and magazine reports was the responsibility of individual women and girls to ensure "a high level of hygiene at all times" (Wright 1982, p. 93) in order to avoid contracting TSS. For example, in only the fourth article to appear about TSS in *The Advertiser* ("Women in Vic." 1981, p.1), there was specified a set of procedures for using tampons in order "to eliminate the risk" of getting TSS. Thus, TSS early on was transformed into a issue of neglect of care for the self, and carelessness on the part of individual women. The solution was to publish the first of many articles outlining steps women should take in order to ensure hygiene of the highest order. The threat of TSS was represented as lying not in the syndrome itself but in ignoring the steps to be taken to avoid it. Consequently, as late as March 1995 Dr. Garland, the Chair of the tampon manufacturer-backed Toxic Shock Syndrome Information Service, is reported as stating "the greatest threat of TSS is ignorance of the illness" (Kerr 1995b, p.26).

However, in the context of her comments Dr. Garland is clearly framing such ignorance as the "fault" of individuals rather than, for example, tampon manufacturers.

Further, such a discourse of taking responsibility for looking after one's own menstrual hygiene, is in keeping with the subtextual frame of menstrual etiquette discussed previously. As Ginsburg (1996) points out, "menstrual etiquette depends most fundamentally for its success upon women's ability and willingness to watch themselves" (p. 373). Thus, women learn to police themselves with respect to both how they "handle" tampons and how they conceal the need for tampons in the first place. Such surveillance represents what Foucault (1975) has termed the gaze which "envelopes, caresses, details, [and] atomizes the most individual flesh" (p.171), resulting in the development of a compliant docile body (Foucault 1977) able to be subject to, object of and even "improved" by discourses of taking responsibility for one's own menstrual hygiene. Relentless self-surveillance of menstrual hygiene and etiquette characterizes the development of such docility in order to attain the "norm" in terms of specific menstrual behaviors. Menstrual etiquette (including self-policing hygiene) is thus normalized: "We fit the pieces together so that they make sense to us and reinforce our ideas about how things work" (Ginsburg 1996, p.367). A subtextual message of the commonsense premise of taking care in handling tampons and "watching" one's menstrual etiquette is thereby developed and sustained.

Around the same time as these self-help directives for avoiding TSS were appearing, *The Australian Women's Weekly* (Munday 1981, p. 13) recorded that "some doctors report a worrying amount of ignorance about just how tampons should be used. One tells how women have come to have examinations still wearing foul tampons that have been left in for days" (p. 13). Not surprisingly, the then Managing Director of Johnson &Johnson, Mr. Colin Bull, in the same article concurred that "personal hygiene and the way a tampon is handled before and during insertion (is) vital." A month later, in March 1981, *The Advertiser* reported that a 15-year-old girl had contracted TSS and stated "she had left one [tampon] in place overnight" (Toxic shock victim No. 4, 1981, p. 6). The same report detailed the National Health and Medical Research Council (NH&MRC) advice about using tampons. While not overtly stated, the implicit assumption was the link between the contraction of TSS by the girl and her ignorance of, or ignoring of, NH&MRC advice. In this way the girl was somehow to "blame" for her contraction of TSS. Like the women alluded to in *The Australian Women's Weekly* article above, she had neglected her personal hygiene responsibilities and had not used tampons "correctly" or in a "normal" way.

However, what these reports assume is that appropriate, objective and accessible information is available both about using tampons and TSS itself. This is questionable. For example, Abraham, Knight, Mira, McNeil and Llewellyn-Jones (1985) report with respect to the information provided about TSS that of:

the young women who decided to use tampons and who sought advice on how to insert the tampon from the manufacturer's pamphlet, one in five found the literature provided was too difficult to follow. (p. 231).

Further, it is interesting to note that women and girls rely upon the manufacturers of tampons themselves for much of their information about tampons and TSS. Delaney et al. (1988), commenting on the role of the manufacturers in providing this information, argue somewhat cynically that this is in fact "education for consumerhood" (p. 108). Referring to the lack of warnings about TSS in the educational materials produced for school and individual consumption by one tampon manufacturer they write:

> not to include information and warnings on the actual books used in the classroom or in the home throws into clear relief the less-than-educational nature of these publications. Selling the product, we are shockingly reminded, is the bottom line (p. 111).

Russell (1993) concurs with respect to the limitations of the material produced to inform women about TSS, alluding to "little ongoing coverage of relative risks, the differences in the types of tampons, and the long delay in getting warning labels to reflect the known risks" (p. 192). Indeed, as we have seen, some of the information disseminated about TSS in popular magazines was confusing and even contradictory, bearing out Russell's (1993) assertion that "too often today....a woman is confronted with a series of confusing, or even contradictory pieces of information about the risks she faces and what she should do about them" (p. 192).

Lupton (1994c) points out that a focus on the individual responsibility for health and the blaming of the victim often "obscures the fact that still very little is known about the causes of the disease and the best way of avoiding it" (p. 85). Although Lupton was alluding to breast cancer, she could just have easily been referring to TSS. Whilst women and girls were being urged to be vigilant and exercise self-surveillance with respect to how they handled a tampon, the fact was that no one could be certain if it was the handling of tampons that was the problem, the tampons themselves" or something else. As Fischer and Skondras (1993) point out:

> it is not certain exactly what is in these products, as there is no legal requirement to disclose the contents of "feminine hygiene products". Contrast this with "beauty products" such as shampoos which by law must have the ingredients listed on the pack. (p. 14)

No matter how vigilant women may be about their own personal hygiene and the way they handle tampons, the question posed by Fischer and Skondras (1993) remains: "Can we rely on the manufacturers of pads and tampons to inform us about these products? It is a billion dollar industry, and companies are not legally bound to give details of ingredients on the packs" (p. 16).

The discursive frame emphasizing individual responsibility for health had the effect of relegating other factors and issues, that is other ways of thinking and talking about TSS, to the margins. These other factors and issues include the fact that tampons undergo no tests for hygiene or safety apart from those tests undertaken by the manufacturers themselves. It is in the interests of powerful societal groups, including manufacturers of tampons, that individual women and their use of tampons, rather than tampons themselves, be framed as the "problem" to be addressed. As Olesen (1986) powerfully reminds us:

> the toxic-shock phenomenon poses critical questions in the definition and construction of the issues....certainly in the case of toxic-shock syndrome, different definitions, predicated on the production of research data and the presumed confounding influences of the mass media of communication were and remain in play. (pp. 57-58)

CONCLUDING COMMENTS

Media representations of TSS, or any other health issue for that matter, are not neutral and value-free. Rather, they both reflect, and in turn construct, certain taken-for-granted assumptions and understandings about reality: "knowledge reflects social, historical and political phenomena" (Collyer 1996, p. 1). Far from just conveying information, media reports can operate to create and sustain certain understandings pertaining to health and health care. Consequently, rather than seeking simply to describe what the media in this study have reported about TSS, the discussion has sought to probe and explore what discursive frames have shaped and framed such reports, and in turn how these reports have operated to sustain dominant discourses about health and health care.

The enabling and constraining effect of three discursive frames—concealment, the scientific/medical and individual responsibility for health—on the way TSS is represented in print-based media articles has been explored. These frames shape what is said about TSS, how it is said and, importantly, what is not said. With respect to what is not said, it was particularly interesting to explore the way TSS has been represented in the media as it touches on the otherwise unmentionable and invisible—menstruation and women's sanitary hygiene. Consequently, the subtextual frame of menstrual etiquette is a powerful influence in the way in which the reporting is shaped. It is as if the articles themselves stand before an omnipresent gaze, a panoptic connoisseur, determining what it is possible to say and not to say. The discourse of concealment highlights the paradox that pervades the reporting about TSS: the ever-present yet normally hidden fact of menstruation, and an associated conspicuous absence of the consumption of sanitary products such as tampons (Ginsburg 1996).

The various discursive frames about TSS reveal competing and often vested interests in its portrayal—those of the tampon manufacturers, health authorities, women and their families affected by TSS, and the legal profession. Gameson's (1990) study of representations of the condom, also an object and topic of discussion that traverses many cultural taboos and which is also associated with a particular etiquette in the way in which it can, and can not, be spoken about, illustrated that:

> meanings proliferate in popular discourse...bitter fights are and have been waged—in courts, in congressional hearing rooms, on television, in scientific journals...to make the condom mean certain things and not others, to associate it with some users and behaviors and disassociate it from others (Gameson 1990, p. 263).

Gameson spoke of "disputed moments" (p. 263) in the understandings created about condoms and it is such disputed moments and their effect in terms of the way in which TSS is represented discursively and subsequently framed, that reveal much about competing interests in the portrayal of TSS. One such disputed moment apparent in ongoing reporting of TSS is the very definition of the syndrome itself.

Yet it is too simplistic to portray media articles as creating a view passively adopted by the readers of those articles. As Kaplan (1992) points out, readers of texts play an active part in determining the viewing positions to be adopted with respect to any one text. She differentiates between the hypothetical reader/spectator position created by the text and the "reading formations" (p. 13) the viewer brings to the text, suggesting that any viewing position adopted is a negotiated one in that there is "delicate negotiation in any textual reception between the hypothetical spectator offered by the novel/film [article] and the reading formations of the reader/viewer" (p. 13). It is a limitation of the analysis offered here that it has only focused on the hypothetical reader/spectator position created by the media articles. Further study is needed on how readers of these articles actually understand and respond to these texts, that is, the negotiated viewing position that is adopted. As Sanders (1988) points out, without the viewer any image or representation is incomplete.

Indeed it is important to recognize that this discussion itself has taken a view. It has created a certain hypothetical reader/spectator position. Readers of this text, like readers of any other, must position themselves with respect to the viewing position created by the discussion. As Frazer (1992) points out, "all too often theorists commit the fallacy of reading 'the' meaning of the text and inferring the ideological effects the text 'must' have on the readers (other than the theorists themselves, of course!)" (p. 186). These limitations aside, the discursive analysis reported here has been a beginning step in enabling an exploration of how certain discourses have the effect of framing debate and routinizing discussion about TSS. In so doing it is hoped that other possibilities and ways of viewing this health issue can emerge, thus challenging and unsettling what otherwise may become everyday, commonsense, taken-for-granted assumptions and understandings about Toxic Shock Syndrome.

SUMMATION

In Chapter 3 the section "Discourse analysis—some concluding comments" explored four stages/features of discourse analysis posited by Parker (1992):

–   The introduction—where the study is positioned in relation to other studies in the field
–   The methodology—in which detail is given about which texts are to be studied and why
–   The analysis—where the data is coded and analyzed under different discourse headings
–   The discussion—where links are made between the findings of the study and other writers and studies in the substantive area under exploration. This includes reflection on the researcher's position in terms of framing the analyses.

The discussion in Chapters 4 and 5 has used a particular study as the vehicle for exploring how one might approach these four stages/features in a research project. Chapter 4 contained detailed examples and explanation about how to prepare a research proposal, addressing the first two stages identified by Parker. Chapter 5 then explored the types of analyses and discussion that might result from this study. In so doing, the aim of these two chapters has been to speak practically in terms of the strategies and struggles involved in carrying out this type of research endeavour. In no way has the aim been to provide a "recipe" to follow. Poststructural and postmodern research is multifaceted and involves many different research approaches and forms of analysis. The example used has been just that—an example to give some insights into the research process used in this particular study. The further readings suggested at the end of this chapter give other examples of reports of research carried out within a postmodern or poststructural frame. It is hoped that you will gain further valuable insights by reading these articles, for I reiterate the point made by Parker (1992)—"Perhaps the best way to get a feel for forms of discourse is to look at how analysts actually deal with texts" (p. 127).

I conclude this section of the book, which has been more practically focused, by returning to the concept of writing for a particular audience. As discussed in Chapter 4, it is important to be aware of the openness or otherwise of funding agencies, editors, editorial boards of journals and publishers to new and different research approaches and analyses such as those afforded by postmodern and poststructural approaches. Rejection of a research submission or a manuscript may often have more to do with understandings of what does, and by implication does not, constitute research and scholarship than with the worthiness of what is submitted. As Silverman and Gubrium (1989) point out:

Grant giving organisations will seek to channel research in particular directions; there is no neutral money, whether one is speaking about the well-meant initiatives of Research Councils and the National Institutes of Health, or the funding schemes of the pharmaceutical and tobacco industries or the war machine. (p. 2)

Thus you may find it useful to write to editors of journals and chairs of funding boards to ascertain their position with respect to research using particular approaches. It is important to recognize and remember that the research process, and even research itself, is discursively framed even though such frames may be so taken for granted as to be invisible.

FURTHER READING

Cheek, J. (1997a). (Con)textualizing Toxic Shock Syndrome: Selected media representations of an emergent health phenomenon 1979-1995, *Health, 1*(2), 183-203.

This article, discussed in depth within the present chapter, explores the way in which four selected Australian print media—one newspaper and three magazines—represent Toxic Shock Syndrome. The discussion explores both descriptive and discursive aspects of the reporting of Toxic Shock Syndrome.

Cheek, J. (1997b). Negotiating delicately: Conversations about health. *Health and Social Care in the Community, 5*(1), 23-27.

This article explores the way in which assumptions about health and health care by health care professionals and their clients, contribute to power relations. It contains an analysis of a conversation between a client and health care professional, and shows the way assumptions about health and health care affect the positions adopted when communicating about health.

Fox, N. (1997). Texts, frames and decisions over discharge from hospital: A deconstruction. *Social Sciences in Health: The International Journal of Research and Practice, 3*(1), 41-51.

Fox describes an ethnographic study in which he deconstructs negotiations between surgeons and patients over discharge from hospital. He focuses on ways in which the interaction between surgeons and patients is framed and the ways in which particular framings "differends" can be seen as acts of power which limit choice and alternative understandings of the situation.

Latimer, J. (1995). The nursing process re-examined: Enrolment and translation. *The Journal of Advanced Nursing, 22*, 213-220.

Latimer excavates the way in which the nursing process has come to be constructed and understood in order to propose "a different way of considering the nursing process" (p. 213). She explores the assumptions and understandings, often so taken for granted as to be invisible, about nurses and nursing practice that are embedded within the concept of the nursing process. She argues that in adopting, and even embracing, the tenets of the nursing process in an effort to professionalize nursing, nurses may have unwittingly, or otherwise, adopted the discourses of others—particularly managerialist devices and techniques. The article troubles the notion that there can be universal modes of how nurses do (or should do) nursing, using the nursing process as the vehicle for discussion.

Lupton, D. (1994c). Femininity, responsibility, and the technological imperative: Discourses on breast cancer in the Australian press. *International Journal of Health Services, 24*(1), 73-89.

Lupton explores Australian print media representations of breast cancer for the period of 1987 to 1990. She identifies three dominant discourses in the reporting of breast cancer: one linking breast cancer to a failure to fulfill "feminine" roles, one relating to medical dominance, and one emphasizing lifestyle factors and individual responsibility for health.

May, C. R. & Purkis, M. E. (1995). The configuration of nurse-patient relationships: A critical view. *Scholarly Inquiry for Nursing Practice, 283-295.*

> May and Purkis trouble the concept of the nurse-patient relationship. They argue that there is little that is self-evident in the forms that nursing has come to take. Rather, what is evident is influenced by various sets of ideas and understandings about nurses and nursing practice—some of which are more pervasive than others. Thus there is a need to uncover and interrogate taken-for-granted aspects of nursing and nursing practice. The article seeks to provide the grounds "on which a reconfiguration of ideas currently employed to conceptualize nurse-patient relationships might be founded".

Thompson, C. & Hirschman, E. (1995). Understanding the socialized body: A poststructuralist analysis of consumer's self-conceptions, body images, and self-care practices. *Journal of Consumer Research, 22,* 139-153.

> This research uses the data from 30 semi-structured interviews to identify ways in which the body of the individual is socialized by dominant discourses about health and beauty. This is discussed in relation to "norms" about the body and in relation to Foucault's notion of the gaze. The authors include detailed description of the research process they undertook.

Weaver, A. (1994). Deconstructing dirt and disease: The case of TB. In M. Bloor & P. Taraborrelli (eds.), *Qualitative Studies in Health and Medicine.* Avebury, UK: Ashgate.

> Weaver explores the binary opposition of clean/dirty evident in ethnographic field notes made about a TB sanatorium. She explores the concept of dirt in relation to disease and argues that the concept of dirt is rooted in power relations. This is evident in the way that different health care professions understand and follow procedures for preventing contamination, thereby confirming the social boundaries between the professions as well as the isolation and observation of those who are viewed as contaminated.

Chapter 6

The Journey Forward

INTRODUCTION

In the last chapter of a book it is customary to reach some sort of "final" statement or conclusion. Such a conclusion usually pulls together the threads of the argument or thesis that have been systematically developed in the preceding pages of the text. Having read such a conclusion, the reader is left with a sense of closure, a sense that a path has been traversed and a certain destination reached.

This conclusion is not like that. In many ways it would be antithetical to the discussion of postmodern and poststructural approaches to attempt to arrive at an end point. Instead, in keeping with the philosophy of these approaches, it is hoped that this final chapter opens up ideas and further avenues for exploration. In so doing, the book will provide you with a way forward, will enable you to pursue your own exploration and analysis of these approaches and allow you to see how they can be applied to research into aspects of nursing and health care. Thus, in many ways this book marks the start of what is hoped will be a journey of discovery for you, the reader. The book has introduced you to some aspects of postmodern and poststructural approaches to research in health care. It is up to each reader to seek out more information as he or she sees fit. All of this is to emphasize that whatever appears in printed form (as with any other form of text) can only ever be a partial and incomplete representation of the reality being presented. There is always more to be said and thought about!

WHERE HAVE WE BEEN?

As the introduction to this chapter has emphasized, this book forms part of a journey of discovery with respect to postmodern and poststructural approaches and their applicability to the nursing and health care arenas. However, reading this book has been a journey in itself, and I think it is a useful exercise at this point to pause in order to reflect where the journey we on which we embarked in reading this book has taken us. Hence the title of this section: "Where have we been?"

The book began by asserting that research in nursing and health care is an evolving process. Part of this process is grappling with issues as fundamental as what the subject matter for "legitimate" research in nursing/health care might be and what appropriate theoretical and methodological frames for such research are. From the outset the discussion promoted the notion of the diversity of approaches to, and areas for, research that are applicable in the nursing/health care arena. Postmodern and poststructural approaches are part of such diversity.

Chapter 1 then moved on to consider some of the issues that have arisen with respect to postmodern and poststructural approaches in research. Not least among these issues was the problem of defining these terms. We noted that discussions of postmodern and poststructural approaches are often fraught with uncertainty about exactly what understanding of these approaches is used. Thus Chapter 1 emphasized the importance of clearly stating the understanding of the words postmodern and poststructural in any piece of research or writing which purports to draw on these approaches. Further, difficulties in clearly delineating postmodern and poststructural approaches from one another were highlighted. "Tidy" definitions, and consequently the "tidy" differentiation of each approach, are not possible as by their very nature postmodern and poststructural approaches resist being placed into tidy, clearly delineated categories.

In response to the issue of the difficulty often associated with providing clear understandings of the way the terms postmodern and poststructural are used, Chapters 2 and 3 of the book explored postmodern and poststructural approaches in order to establish working definitions that could inform the discussion throughout the text. Indeed, the project of the entire book could be considered as establishing working understandings both of these approaches themselves and the ways in which they can inform research in nursing and health care. In both Chapters 2 and 3, the works of key theorists in the area were considered and used to illustrate the points being made.

Chapters 2 and 3 also gave examples of research that have used postmodern and/or poststructural frames. This set the scene for the next two chapters which spoke in a more practical way about actually proposing and doing research using these approaches. By closely exploring the genesis and subsequent implementation of a research project which involved the discursive analysis of aspects of the reporting of health/illness by the media, Chapters 4 and 5 provided insights into some of the issues to be considered and problems to be grappled with when conceptualizing such research.

Another issue discussed in Chapter 1 was the question of the applicability of these approaches in informing the practical reality of the health care setting. This issue has formed a thread that has run through all the chapters of the book, namely, consideration of the question posed in Chapter 1—can postmodern and poststructural approaches influence practice or are they merely esoteric? Many of the examples of research studies and findings used in Chapters 2 and 3 were chosen specifically because they highlighted how these approaches can inform practice.

The subject matter in the examples has ranged from the organization of ward rounds and case note documentation to the ways in which popular media shape, and are in turn shaped by, dominant assumptions and understandings of health and health care. We have seen that postmodern and poststructural research approaches can illuminate and challenge aspects of health care and health care delivery, ranging from more micro levels of analysis such as that of individual ward settings, to the macro focus of societal representation of health care issues.

Chapter 1 highlighted the fact that much of the criticism of these approaches in terms of their apparent inability to influence practice stems from assumptions about the research that is "deliverable"; or what Gouldner (1971) termed the "background assumptions" about what a research project and its product should be. In particular, the notion of the immediacy of the applicability of research findings was explored. It was noted that in the climate of economic rationalism that so pervades contemporary Western society, immediate and often quantifiable benefits of research are demanded. In such a mood it is easy to overlook the need for what Porter (1997) termed the basic research upon which more applied and instrumentally orientated research can build. Purkis (1994) extends this point when she writes:

> Pressure to provide answers is understood within the context of this article as a linguistic device widely employed in the literature for legitimating research efforts, that is, in response to an approach to the field of study where research is understood as fulfilling a "need" to inform practice. (p. 15)

Thus Purkis is questioning the assumption that research must fulfil a "need" (either spoken or unspoken) to inform practice in the first place. In so doing she is challenging understandings about what research is for and what outcomes of research might and "should" be.

Once we begin thinking, speaking and writing within postmodern and poststructural frames, many assumed understandings in the research process are open to scrutiny and challenge. thus, the book has taken us on a journey which began with thge posing of two major questions: what are postmodern and poststructural approaches, and can these approaches be used in research to inform the practical realities of the world of the health care setting? These issues have been explored at length.

In addition, the way in which research which draws on these approaches can be developed and carried out has been integral to the discussion about these two issues. At times, the journey we have taken has led us over some rocky theoretical ground, with many potential paths to follow. No easy answers present themselves to the questions and issues that arise. However, we have been able to map out some guiding principles which serve both to inform our explorations and to avoid the discussion becoming bogged down in the mire of theoretical and methodological ambiguity, vagueness, and assumed understandings about the nature, conduct and purpose of the research endeavour.

I wish to conclude this discussion of our journey by offering a cautionary note. It is timely to reiterate a theme that has permeated the discussion throughout the book, that is, that postmodern and poststructural approaches should in some way be viewed as privileged, mandatory, or as replacing other approaches to research. Rather, this book suggests that postmodern and poststructural approaches have a place in nursing and health care research along with other theoretical perspectives and methodological approaches. It is not an either/or situation. Instead, it is more a matter of enabling and allowing a variety of research approaches and theoretical frames to inform research and subsequent knowledge development in the nursing and health care areas. What Rosenau (1994) asserts with respect to the futility of adopting polemic positions regarding "modern" as opposed to "postmodern" sociology, applies equally to the futility of attempting to adopt polemic positions with respect to "modern" and "postmodern" approaches to research. She writes:

> I would like to argue that the confrontation between modern and postmodern sociology is fruitless. First, there are no "entities" as such—modern sociology and post-modern sociology. Both are heterogeneous collections of views that overlap at the edges and are not mutually exclusive, neat, clear categories. Second, we may have here a case of different competences in different spheres. The knowledge claims of each are potentially adequate and appropriate in different circumstances and given various purposes. (p. 96)

It is not a case of attempting to replace one grand narrative with another!

At all times, the rationale for choosing a particular research approach rather than other possibilities must stated clearly. The strengths and limitations of the various approaches must be recognized, as must the role that theoretical and methodological frames play in shaping research understandings, research undertakings, and conclusions reached from that research. Postmodern and poststructural approaches, like any other approach to research, represent certain views of reality. Put another way, postmodern and poststructural approaches themselves are discursive constructions, drawing on certain knowledge claims to give them presence. Thus, they are open to the same sort of challenge and scrutiny as any other theoretical frame.

WHERE ARE WE?

The previous section in this chapter provided you with an overview of where the discussion of the book has led us so far. Where does this leave us now, then? Hopefully it leaves us in a position of wanting to know more about these approaches and the research that has arisen, and can arise, from them. The further readings that have been suggested at the end of each chapter, including this one, should enable you to continue your explorations. This book is just a beginning, and a very brief beginning at that!

It is also hoped that as a result of the exploration of these approaches, you are beginning to question and explore assumptions and understandings implicit within your practice area and/or research that previously you may have taken for granted. All of this involves the development of reflexivity on the part of the reader and/or researcher.

Porter (1993) notes that the development of reflexivity "entails researchers viewing their own beliefs in the same fashion as they view those held by their subjects" (p. 141). The research process itself, in that it is a form of text that is discursively constituted, thus becomes a focus of the reflexive researcher. Apparent "givens" such as understandings of reliability and validity, or what does or does not constitute research, are opened up to scrutiny. The same is true for the form that research texts take. Porter (1993) ably demonstrates reflexivity in action in his exploration of why certain journal editorial boards and manuscripts reviewers reject the use of the word "I" in papers submitted for publication. He argues that there is no logical reason why manuscripts using the first person, that is, "I", should be viewed as less scholarly than those which use the passive voice. Rather, such reasons stem from largely unexplored assumptions about what constitutes "good" and/or appropriate scholarly writing, which in turn, often arises from the discursive frame of the supposed disinterested objectivity that the passive voice purports to represent. Porter (1993) asserts that "the academic text is just as much the result of convention and contrivance as any other cultural artifact. We can not take the conventionality of texts for granted; their language needs to be treated as problematic" (p. 142).

Such reflexivity and the questioning it promotes also applies to enacted texts (Jacobson & Jacques, 1997); that is, the field notes, observations, interview transcripts and so forth that purport to represent aspects of the reality under scrutiny by a researcher. In other words, we need to look at the texts themselves, rather than assume texts are simply neutral conveyors of information. Any representation of reality which takes the form of empirical materials and data collected in a research undertaking will only ever represent partial aspects of the reality being studied. Further, how those aspects are represented will be shaped and influenced by the assumptions and frames that researchers bring with them and impose on the research process. Thus empirical materials themselves must be scrutinized for what they reveal about the reality portrayed. Empirical materials are the textual record of what has been observed, studied and subsequently "found". As such they are open to the same scrutiny as any other form of text. Hertz (1996) captures the idea of looking at texts well when she writes:

> Through personal accounting researchers should become more aware of how their own positions and interests are imposed at all stages of the research process—from the questions they ask to those they ignore, from whom they study to whom they ignore, from problem formation to analysis, representation and writing—in order to produce less distorted accounts of the social world. (p. 5)

Reflexivity also brings into scrutiny the notion of the research "field", both in terms of what the field is, and how that field is represented in the research text. The field for any particular research endeavour is not out there waiting to be described by researchers. Rather, the field is a construction of the researcher. It is the researcher who defines the field for a particular study and who then goes about constructing that field by the collection of research data. In turn, the role of the researcher is, at least in part, constructed by the understanding of the field in play. Turner (1989) points out that Foucault's work, for example, provides "us with an analysis of the forces that produce "the field"—both the lie of the land itself, and the shaping of the eye that surveys it" (p. 17).

Subsequently Jacobson and Jacques (1997) discuss the effect of destabilizing the field, that is, challenging the notion of a fixed, stable field of study. When reporting on the field for a study looking at how the social space of nursing has been, and is, constructed and maintained, they note:

> The object of the research is not the nurse but the lens through which the nurse is represented. The goal is not one of better understanding what is really going on but one of understanding how any construction of the real is influenced by the relationships of power through which the structure of social reality has been produced and is maintained, often in seemingly mundane ways. (p. 54)

Thus, the field itself can be explored to expose the ways in which the field is both constructed and positioned by the researcher, and which in turn constructs and positions the researcher. Hence Turner (1989) defines the field in the following way:

> It constitutes, shall we say, an attitude towards their "clients" needed by agents of social control, a framing of the life of actual or potential subjects, a point of view which will force an intersection of the interests of the inquirer and the life of the subject. (p. 14)

Postmodern and poststructural approaches enable the development of a reflexivity that can challenge and open up to scrutiny otherwise closed and taken-for-granted aspects of both the research process and nursing and health care practice. Far from being nihilistic and entirely destructive, as Eagleton (1983) suggests when stating that these approaches allow "you to drive a coach and horses through everybody else's beliefs while not saddling you with the inconvenience of having to adopt any yourself" (p. 144), postmodern and poststructural approaches offer new and different perspectives on the practice realm. In offering such perspectives, there is no claim to the last word or definitive answers. Rather, there is a desire to "become more reflexive about the ways that situated knowers and knowns influence the production of inevitably perspective-dependent knowledge" (Jacobson & Jacques, 1997, p. 56).

A reflexive approach can expose what we are and offer other possibilities for what we might be. In this way it may be possible to "avoid both the positivism of the window and the nihilism of the mirror" (Turner, 1989, p. 25) for, as Turner (1989) points out, in refusing what we are or what is (Foucault 1980), there is a risk that we may "render ourselves homeless by an act of will" (Turner, p. 20).

I wish to conclude this section on the development of a reflexive approach to analyses of aspects of reality, including those of nursing and health care, by referring you to Exhibits 6.1 and 6.2. These exhibits outline work currently being carried out which challenges, in a reflexive manner, taken-for-granted aspects of health care delivery. One of the studies analyzes the effect of critical pathways on the practice of nurses. Thus it focuses on the management of nursing work. The other study explores the way in which pain is understood and managed by nurses. Hence, it explores a central aspect of nursing care and practice. The subject matter of these research endeavours highlights the applicability of postmodern and poststructural approaches to the practice realm. The practice realm itself is exposed as a set of beliefs that "are neither self-evident, necessary, nor in correspondence with any one demonstrable Real" (Jacobson & Jacques, 1997, p. 55).

Exhibit 6.1   Outline of a study being carried out by Lynne Barnes, PhD candidate, University of South Australia to explore "the use of critical pathways by registered nurses in an acute ward of a private metropolitan hospital in South Australia." This exhibit was prepared by Lynne.

CONTEXT. My study is an exploration of the effects of critical pathways on the practice of nurse clinicians in a metropolitan, South Australian hospital. Critical pathways have emerged as a multi-disciplinary strategy for coordinating clinical care in the context of an increased focus on efficiency, effectiveness and competition in Australian health and social policy.

In a discussion paper "The issue of critical pathways in Australia" Gibb and Banfield (1996:43) stated that: "... clinical staff are being beguiled into accepting strategies and thinking more akin to corporate business interest [sic] revolving around the efficient operation of health care facilities, than their own discipline."

This notion of clinicians being "beguiled" stimulated an interest in exploring the effects of the "strategies and thinking" of dominant discourses, such as economic and managerial, on the practice of clinicians, through an interrogation of the implementation of critical pathways.

I began the study by exploring the positioning of critical pathways within the literature and tracing their lineage back to engineering where they were developed to more effectively plan and control complex work. The concept was adopted by the New England Medical Centre (USA) in the 1980s where it is described as a tool for use within the case management model of managed care delivery. However, although the "tool" is reported as being multi-disciplinary the literature describing its use is almost exclusively nursing.

METHOD. In conducting the study I use ethnographic techniques to examine the clinical use of critical pathways in order to generate a text for analysis using a form of discourse analysis informed primarily by the writings of Michel Foucault. Text generation is initially in the form of "field notes" which are a collection of writings (re)presenting my interaction with "the field" on various levels.

Text is generated from the literature, meetings with nurses, and notes taken whilst observing clinical practice. Interviews with clinicians help to position and interpret the text generated from observations and from the clinicians'' recording of patients' "case notes".

Simultaneous with the process of generating field notes is a form of reflexive interaction with the text in order to give attention to the socio-political forces within which it is positioned. As an ongoing process all data is assembled, read and re-read to gain a sense of its textual, contextual and inter-textual dimensions. This process is reflexive with all areas of data collection and analysis: each influencing and reconstructing the other.

The analysis is predicated on the notion of its objective being to expose the network of discourses which shape the implementation of critical pathways by the nurses participating - not to produce a problem solving theory. Thus the text produced by the analysis is not **the** end, or even **an** end, but part of an ongoing process - a text which positions the reader as having a role and function in its (re)construction and in the on going process of nursing subjectivity.

OBSTACLES. Although the study has been facilitated at management level of the hospital which is the study site, where support for nursing research is promoted, at the clinical level my initial experience was different.

The focus of clinicians was on "getting the work done" and in that respect participation in a research project was seen as an extra burden. Even the most interested of the nurse clinicians whom I addressed in my initial call for participants expressed reservations about her ability to incorporate my presence in an already full time frame. Because of these expressed concerns I became overly anxious about being "in the way" and initially this affected my role as observer on the ward. As time progressed and my presence on the ward became more "commonplace" both I and the clinicians became more relaxed and the "obstacle" reduced.

A further obstacle related to my role of observer was the nurses perceptions of "not being good enough". It was of considerable concern to me that nurses were reluctant to participate and expressed the need to modify their practice to present a more "favourable" impression. I needed to spend considerable time reassuring prospective participants that I was not there to "judge" their standard of practice. Again this obstacle did reduce with time and my presence in the field formed part of my reflexive engagement with my field notes.

PRACTICAL OUTCOMES. The anticipated practical outcomes of this study derive from the provision of a place from which nurse clinicians can critically engage with the "strategies and thinking" of the dominant discourses alluded to by Gibb and Banfield (1996:43).

Nurses, (predominantly women in a role seen as subservient to medicine) are often positioned as disempowered or "victims" - not informed: but "beguiled". Whilst such theoretical constructs have a consciousness raising effect which may be beneficial, they also have the tendency to perpetuate their own truth. In contrast, the text generated by this study, enables a reflexive questioning of that which is taken-for-granted. Thus, rather than being "beguiled", nurses can resist: developing strategies and thinking in accord with their own practice and discursive frame.

This outcome is achieved by using the analysis to interrogate the strategies involved in the interpretation and evaluation of critical pathways in the local context by challenging the taken-for-granted nature of transparent concepts (such as efficiency and effectiveness) and the dominant discourses within which they are positioned. Thus, by making the "taken-for-granted" problematic and using discourse as the unit of analysis, the analysis is positioned to examine the power relations enacted in the practice setting. This allows an interrogation of the notion of clinicians being "beguiled" (Gibb and Banfield, 1996) and an examination of the degree, if any, of their complicity in the process. Also, by juxtaposing competing discursive practices, political, social and cultural boundaries are disrupted and the potential provided for their redrawing. This act of "(re)territorialisation" provides the space for resistance by nurse clinicians.

Reference:

Gibb, H. and Banfield, M. (1996). The issue of critical paths in Australia: Where are they taking us? *Nursing Inquiry*, 3, 36-44.

Exhibit 6.2:   Outline of a study being carried out by Kay Price, PhD candidate, University of South Australia to "explore the way in which nurses construct pain." This exhibit was prepared by Kay.

CONTEXT. I want to explore how it is that nurses construct understandings of pain and the management of that pain for adult persons having elective surgery. In particular I want to focus on how this construction shapes nurses" and adult persons" subjectivity. Like Weedon (1987), I refer to subjectivity as the conscious and unconscious thoughts and emotions of an individual, the sense of self, and the ways of understanding the self in relation to the world. Subjectivity, or the subject position of nurses, is important to focus on because nurses" subjectivity will be different within different understandings of meanings and in each different meaning there will be different political implications for nurses and nursing.

I believe that nursing and medicine organise and structure "how to care" differently (Price 1996). For me, this means that nursing and medicine will approach "pain" and the management of that pain from different perspectives. Yet, when reviewing how "pain" is represented in nursing and medical literature, I contend that there is much for nursing and nurses to be concerned about.

It is my argument that pain has been made the focus of attention which overlooks the very object of nursing"s focus—the person. Nurses never encounter "pain" without there being a person or persons involved.

In literature written by nurses on the topic of pain and/or pain management, nurses have (overtly or covertly) constructed their arguments/views within the implicit understanding and meaning of pain as represented by scientific-medical discourse (Price and Cheek 1996a). Such a representation reports that pain results from tissue damage (actual or potential) from which it is assumed that "pain is what the subject [patient] says hurts" (Bishop, 1959). It has been taken for granted that this representation of pain was appropriate for both nursing and medicine.

Scientific-medical discourse promotes a politics of sameness in relation to pain and the management of pain for persons having surgery (Price and Cheek 1996b). This is particularly evident in literature which promotes institutionalising pain management for example, as a way to overcome the perceived problem of undertreatment of pain. I do not discount the "reality" of pain. Rather, I suggest that there are many different ways in which to view this "reality". Institutionalising pain management not only negates the view that pain and its management means different things to different people, but it also negates the political struggles which exist in hospital settings and thereby potentially marginalises and silences nursing"s contribution to care outcomes.

My theoretical context emphasises that language, power and knowledge organise and structure meanings of events such as "pain" and that the subject position of persons will be different within different meanings. I have been drawn to the writings of Jacques Derrida and Michel Foucault to provide the theoretical context in which my analysis occurs. I am aware that I am creating texts for analysis, that my research is a text, and that my thesis will be a text. This requires of me to be reflexive, and in so doing establish my integrity as researcher and author of these texts. I am inviting the reader to continue and develop my argument.

METHOD. Brewer"s (1994) description of an ethnographic methodology is that which I am using in my research. While ethnography has been subject to criticism, and different approaches to ethnography have been adopted in different areas, guided by different concerns (Atkinson and Hammersley 1994), I believe it to be a most appropriate methodology for generating texts for postmodern/poststructural critiques. In such critiques, the experience of being a person is captured in the notion of subjectivity. To understand the processes through which a person is made subject, or how nurses" subjectivity is constituted and operates, requires a researcher being part of the social world of the research setting. This is what ethnography offers.

I use a triangulation of research methods—observation; interviewing of nurses and persons having surgery; and, collection of relevant documentation—from which I assemble texts for analysis. My intent is to interrogate the "reality" produced in these texts and those from literature, to show how the subjectivity of nurses and persons having surgery is shaped with respect to the way nurses construct understandings of pain and the management of that pain. Also how pain is premised on certain understandings. For example, in one of my chapters I want to show how pain is, and has been, institutionally constructed to explain the powerful effects of organisational strategies in privileging a particular meaning of pain and thus establishing the boundaries of being a nurse. To do this I will analyse texts such as: hospital information brochures; centralised hospital services; experiences; policy and procedure documents; memorandums; admission procedures; information booklets; and, nursing interactions with persons having surgery.

OBSTACLES. Before ethical approval was granted by the institutional ethics committee where I wanted to conduct my research, my supervisor and I were invited to speak to my proposal. While an unusual practice, the invitation was extended as committee members acknowledged that they had received few proposals of the kind I had submitted. We experienced resistance from some members of the ethics committee who voiced concerns about; the research methods of observation and interviewing resulting in a "biased" view being projected by nurses (a critique of qualitative methods in general); my research having the potential to lead to conflict between nurses and doctors; and, doubts about the usefulness of my study as the hospital had what was considered an effective Acute Pain Service and as a consequence the role of nurses had changed.

The nature of these concerns reflects certain views about research and also raises to question the role of ethics committees. None-the-less, my proposal was approved and I was able to commence my research. Where I had initially intended to observe nurses (who had given their consent) in their interactions with adult persons having surgery, I realised that I would have to firstly obtain the consent of the adult person who was involved in this interaction. As a consequence of my understanding of the *Privacy Act,* 1988 I could only review case-notes of those adult persons who had given me their consent to do so. Also, I had indicated in my ethics proposal that I would only approach adult persons having surgery to consent to participate in my study before their surgery. With the advent of a pre-admission clinic in the hospital, for awhile there I thought that mine would be the first PhD thesis written from the passage way of the ward in that it was difficult to secure the consent of adult persons given all the above issues.

Having secured the consent of adult persons I was then presented with ethical concerns of sitting in a ward bay of six beds observing one consenting adult person yet not having the consent of the other persons in the bay nor all the hospital personnel or relatives/friends who interacted with these persons. In consultation with the senior nurse it was agreed that so my research could proceed, I did not require the consent of all persons in the bay as long as I had the consent of the adult person I was documenting observations of in my field notes (and would be interviewing), and the nurses in the ward who would interact with this person. In doing this there remains ethical concerns particularly with regard to determining what empirical materials I can utilise in assembling texts for analysis.

PRACTICAL OUTCOMES. I do not conceive of nurses and nursing as being oppressed. Nurses exercise power, yet the exercise of this power may bring about, even contribute to, outcomes that may be not only undesirable for persons having surgery but also make nurses subject to the control of others (eg: medicine) (Price, 1996). Nurses shape their own subjectivity. In relation to pain and the management of pain for persons having surgery, the meaning of pain that nurses privilege will constitute their subjectivity and in turn, in their interactions with persons having surgery constitute the subjectivity of this individual. If nurses privilege the knowledge and language of "others" (in this case, the scientific-medical representation of pain) rather than the knowledge and language of nursing, how do nurses promote the practice of nursing? Nurses are not passive, they area active persons and have the choice when positioning themselves in relation to various discourses. Devaluing the potential of nursing to contribute in its own right to care outcomes in pain management for people having surgery sets up the very conditions that mitigate against nursing"s claim as a discipline. Indeed, against other disciplinary groups involvement in the care of persons having surgery as well.

Pain is a discursive construction within which exists the interplay of other discursive constructions (Price & Cheek 1996a). Both understandings of pain and pain management are textually mediated. Exploring and exposing how nurses construct pain is not to imply that scientific-medical discourse, and the technologies that derive from it, have no place in understanding and managing pain. Rather, it suggests that there are a number of different ways in which to view the reality of pain and the management of that pain, not just one.

My study opens up the possibility for reconceptualising taken-for -granted aspects of practice, eg: pain management and the taken-for granted understandings of pain. This will also trouble other aspects of taken-for granted practice too. As well, it examines whether nurses are complicit in devaluing nursing in care outcomes in pain management for persons having surgery. A complicity that may bring about intended results at the micro or local level of practice yet, in the larger schema, the macro-level (socio-political-legal arena), actually serves to perpetuate the marginalisation and silencing of nursing and nurses. In using the substantive topic of pain and pain management, my findings I believe are useful for illustrating how nurses can resit "being complicit".

References:

Atkinson, P. & Hammersley, M. (1994). Ethnography and Participant Observation. In N.K. Denzin & Y. S. Lincoln (eds.), *Handbook of Qualitative Research* (pp. 248 - 261). Thousand Oaks: Sage Publications.

Bishop, G.H. (1959). Personal communication cited in H. K. Beecher (ed.), *Measurement of subjective responses.* New York: Oxford University Press.

Brewer, J.D. (1994). The Ethnographic Critique Of Ethnography: Sectarianism In The RUC. *Sociology, 28*(1): 231 - 244.

Price, K. (1996). Nursing, pain and pain management. *Nursing Inquiry, 4,* 72-73

Price, K. & Cheek, J. (1996a). Pain as a discursive construction. *Social Sciences in Health, 2*(4): 211 - 217

Price, K & Cheek, J. (1996b) Exploring the nursing role in pain management from a post-structuralist perspective. *Journal of Advanced Nursing, 24,* 899 - 904.

Weedon, C. (1987). *Feminist practices and post-structuralist theory.* New York: Blackwell.

THE JOURNEY FORWARD

The book that you are about to finish reading has been an attempt to create a "writerly" text as opposed to a "readerly" text.

> A "readerly" text assumes a passive reader seeking to understand an author's intentions. It is the opposite of a "writerly" text that is purposely vague, open to many interpretations, and deliberately encouraging the reader to rewrite the contents of the text. (Rosenau, 1992, p. 167)

As a "writerly" text, the book has attempted to engage readers reflexively in the discussion. In so doing it has offered challenges to readers to explore their own taken-for-granted assumptions about research and the health arena.

You may remember that the preface of this book indicated to you that the impetus to write this book stemmed, at least in part, from my own and others' experience of rejection of funding applications and papers sent to journals for publication. Such rejection led me to question the assumptions that were being made about research, scholarship and the "product" of research and scholarship. This questioning enabled me to understand more clearly what was going on in terms of discursive constructions of research and scholarship, and to therefore be better able to target journals, other publishers and funding schemes which are less rigidly bound in discourse. In the same way, I hope that this book increases the reader's ability to target appropriate audiences for their research and scholarship which draws on these approaches.

Postmodern and poststructural analyses of nursing and health care *can* be published, *can* be used in research and *can* influence practice.

Giroux (1992) has promoted what he terms "border crossing" (p. 22) in order to create "borderlands" (p. 22) or "alternate public spaces" (p. 22) where it is possible to rewrite "histories, identities and learning possibilities" (p. 30). This book has promoted the crossing of borders in order to move into and to create new spaces from which to view and research aspects of nursing and health care. Postmodern and poststructural approaches to research open up new territories, pushing beyond the constraints of the discursive borders of taken-for-granted understandings of research and of health care. As in any journey of exploration and discovery, the way forward is fraught with dangers and difficulties. Nevertheless, the potential offered by such a journey for opening up and rewriting histories, identities and research possibilities (to paraphrase Giroux) is enormous, and well worth the risk and the unsettling effect of challenging aspects of reality we have come to take for granted. This book has been a small part of such a journey forward. I hope that it encourages readers to continue on this journey of exploration.

FURTHER READINGS

Cheek, J. (1996). Taking a view: Qualitative research as representation. *Qualitative Health Research, 6*(4), 459-507.

> In this article, I challenge the idea that qualitative research produces an "authentic" version of reality. I argue instead that any research approach is textually mediated: that it encodes assumptions and values about the social world. This affects both the material gathered and the way it is represented. The article explores these assumptions and the way they position the reader of qualitative research.

Hertz, R. (1996). Introduction: Ethics, reflexivity and voice. *Qualitative Sociology, 19*(1), 3-9.

> Hertz explores three issues surrounding ethnographic research: those of ethics, reflexivity and voice. Of particular interest is her contention that a reflexive ethnographer recognizes the "location of self" (p. 5) within the research process. This implies a recognition of how the researcher's social location and interests shape the research process. This is reflected in the use of voice, which is the way authors choose to represent themselves within the ethnography.

Porter, S. (1993). Nursing research conventions: Objectivity or obfuscation? *Journal of Advanced Nursing, 18,* 137-143.

> Porter attacks the use of the third person in academic writings, arguing that it is based on mistaken assumptions about the possibility of obtaining "objective" knowledge. He argues instead, that all knowledge can be seen as arising from a process of social construction. Given this, he calls for reflexivity in nursing research: for nursing researchers to position themselves in relation to their research topic and approach.

Purkis, M. E. (1994). Representations of action: Reorientating field studies in nursing practice. In P. Chinn (ed.), *Advances in Methods of Inquiry for Nursing* (pp. 13-31). Gaithsburg: Aspen.

> Purkis problematizes the relationship between the researcher and the field in practice-based nursing research. She argues that the field is not separate from the researcher, but is a "lifeworld" in which all participants, including the researcher, enact practices together. She draws on, and critiques, a number of field studies in developing her argument.

Turner, R. (1989). Deconstructing the field. In Gubrium J. & Silverman, D. (Eds.), *The Politics of Field Research: Sociology Beyond Enlightenment* (pp.13 -29). London: Sage.

> Turner addresses Foucauldian critiques of the field, particularly focusing on the ways in which the "situatedness" of knowledge, and of the power relations evident in the creation of knowledge, undermine notions of a value-free and objective research field.

Appendix A

1.   **Please indicate '✓' in the relevant box below:**

ARC Small   Internal Research
Grant Only   **✔**   Development Grant
                                                            Only

          Closing date   **Closing date**
        15 September 1995   **13 October 1995**

2.   **If your application is for**   **I**   3.   **Please indicate in the box the**   **3**
      an ARC Small   **panel number(s) of the most**
      Grant, please indicate in   **appropriate panel(s)**
      the box whether
      your application is: **by which your application**
      Initial – I or Renewal – R   **will be assessed:**

4. **Project title:**

Maximum 38 characters per line (4 lines). Do not use quotation marks
Constructing Toxic Shock Syndrome: Selected Australian Print based media
representations of Toxic Shock Syndrome from 1979-1995

5. Total funds requested:

1996	1997 (ARC Small Grants only)	1998 (ARC Small Grants only)
$16,490		

Socio economic Objectives	13000	100%	Field of Research Classification	11000	100%

6. Chief Investigators (see Guidelines)

	1	2	3
a. Title (eg. Prof, A/Prof, Dr) Initials and surname	A/Prof J Cheek		
b. Full address	Faculty of Nursing Telephone Facsimile E-mail	Telephone Facsimile E-mail	Telephone Facsimile E-mail
c. Name of Dept/School/Other (please indicate which)	Faculty of Nursing		
d. Year of birth			
e. Highest academic qualification	PhD		
f. Sex (please tick box)	M ☐ F ✓	M ☐ F ☐	M ☐ F ☐
g. Average working days per month to be devoted to the project			

7. Key Words – Give up to three Key Words to describe the subject area of this proposal:

Toxic Shock Syndrome	Media	Representation

8. Summary of Project

Write a summary, in no more than eight lines, intelligible to a lay reader, of the aims of the research, the expected outcomes and the overall significance. Do not use quotation marks. (Each line allows 54 characters including spaces)

> The way in which the print based media, including popular magazines, represents health issues, influences and shapes societal attitudes towards illness and understandings of health risk. This study explores the way in which a relatively new health phenomenon, Toxic Shock Syndrome, has been represented in Australian print based media from 1979-1995. In so doing it will, by textual analysis of articles pertaining to Toxic Shock Syndrome, uncover changing and different representations of Toxic Shock Syndrome and their effect on perceptions of Toxic Shock Syndrome and related women's health issues and risks.

9. Support

a. Are you applying for support for this or a closely-related project in 1996 from any other source?

Yes ☐ No ☑

If Yes, specify which agency

_____

Note: Please ensure you enter full details in Section 15

b. Have you applied for any of the four ARC Research Fellowships?

Yes ☐ No ☑

c. This question relates to applications for:

Internal Research Development Grants only

Do you intend to apply for support for this project from other sources in the future?

Yes ☐ No ☐

If yes, please specify year(s), source, eg, ARC, GIRD,
Industry

10. Work Experiments

a. Does the work proposed involve research with human subjects?

Yes ☐ No ☑

d. Does the work proposed involve experiments in which there is preparation or use of recombinant nucleic acids constructed in vitro from sources which do not ordinarily recombine genetic information?

Yes ☑ No ☐

b. Does the work proposed involve animal experimentation

Yes ☐ No ☑

c. Does the work proposed involve the use of ionising radiation?

Yes ☐ No ☑

e. Does the work proposed involve the use of toxic sugstances?

Yes ☑ No ☐

11. Chief Investigator Information

If any Chief Investigator is associated with a Special Research Centre or Cooperative Research Centre, supporting documentation is required.

For each Chief Investigator, indicate the following:

a.   Source of salary and % from each source

1	2	3
Associate Professor Julianne Cheek University of SA 100%		

b.   Other major research programs being undertaken or supervised by the Chief Investigator

1	2	3
Analysing the Triage process and its impact on the provision of care and resources allocation in a community nursing context in South Australia *Women and information: The women's information switchboard of South Australia Knowing what needs to be known: A consumer asthma study *Quality use of medications by registered nurses		
Average days per month spent 12 on these programs		

* Completing at the end of 1995

<table>
<tr><td colspan="2">
Other Participants
12. Provide details of the Associate Investigators.
     List: *name
            *organisation
            *highest qualification
            *date conferred
            *conferring institution
            *involvement in the project
            (average days/month)
</td></tr>
</table>

Other Participants

12. Provide details of the Associate Investigators.
    List: *name   *date conferred
           *organisation   *conferring institution
           *highest qualification   *involvement in the project
                                         (average days/month)

13. **What technical and other staff (other than those requested) will be available to assist with this project?**
    Indicate the level of their involvement in the project (average days/month).

14. Budget Information

Detailed budget items	Priority	Amount Requested		
		1996	**1997** ARC Small Grants only	**1998** ARC Small Grants only
Personnel				
Research Assistant Step 1 ($29,554)				
Phase 1 - 0.6x4 months x 29,554	A	**$5912.00**		
Phase 2 - 0.4x5 months x 29,554	A	**$4925.00**		
Phase 3 - 0.2x3 months x 29,554		**$1478.00**		

		$12,315.00		
+ 13.2 Oncosts		**$1,625.00**		

		$13,940.00		
Clerical Assistant				
20 hours x $15.00	A	**$300.00**		

Maintenance				
Costs associated with locating and obtaining articles	A	**$2,000.00**		
Printing	A	**$200.00**		
General Photocopying (eg of drafts)		**$50.00**		

Financial summary

Support requested	Personnel $	Equipment $	Maintenance $	Travel $	Vessel $	Other $	Total $
1996	14,240	2,000	25				16,490.00
1997 (ARC Small Grants)							
1998 (ARC Small Grants)							

15. Total support for this project or a closely related project

List the support received, requested or to be requested from your own organisation and all other sources, excluding this application				
Name of organisation and title of project	1993 $	1994 $	1995 $	Requested 1996

16. Total support for all other projects

List the support received, requested or to be requested from any funding source. Continue on a separate sheet if necessary.				
Name of organisation and title of project	1993 $	1994 $	1995 $	Re'ted 1996
Quality Industry and learning Links (DEET) Issues arising from undergraduate nurse's assessments - The clinician's view. A grounded case study.	$5,202.56 (gained)			
Quality industry and Learning Links (DEET) The notion of success: An exploration of what constitutes a successful industrial placement for undergraduate nursing students	$9,348.00 (gained)			
Centre for Nursing Research Specialist Nurse practitioners - Who are they and why are they there?		$5,000.00 (gained)		
University of South Australia Identifying critical aspects of nursing for aged and extended care		$17,500.00 (gained)		
University of South Australia The health care experience of newly arrived migrant women		$17,500.00 (gained)		
Department of Heath, Housing, Local Government and Community Services Knowing what needs to be known: A community asthma medication study		$71,534.00 (gained)		
Department of health , Housing, Local Government and community Services Quality use of medications by registered nurses		$188, 744.00 (gained)		
Australian Research Council (Small grants scheme) Masculinity and men's health: An exploration and analysis of Australian print based media representations of men's health over a 12 month period			$10,000.00 (gained)	

17. Average number of working days per month to be devoted to all projects to be undertaken in 1997 (including this project)

| 1st Chief Investigator | 12 days | 2nd Chief Investigator | __ days | 3rd Chief Investigator | __ days |

18. Commencement/Completion day of project

Has the project started? Yes ☐ No ☑   If No, when will it start?

How long will you need ARC support?   1 Years   How long will this project take?   1 Years

19. Will there be any research or honours students working on the project?

If Yes, state the number in each case   Yes ☐ No ☑

16. Total support for all other projects (cont)

Name of organisation and title of the project	1993	1994	1995	Requested 1996
Migrant Health Services The health care experiences of newly arrived migrant women			$45,000.00 (gained)	
University of South Australia Women and information: The women's information switchboard of South Australia			$13,000.00 (gained)	
Health Enhancement Research Grant Scheme (SAHC) Analysing the triage process and its impact on the provision of care and resource allocation in a community nursing context in South Australia			$14,827.00 (gained)	
University of South Australia CATHIE monies (DEET) Open learning package on information literacy	$3,000.00 (gained)			
Innovation Grants Scheme: University of South Australia Finding Out: Using Information			$5,000.00 (gained)	

Committee for the Advancement of University Teaching (DEET) Using Hypertext to Promote Flexible Learning in a Graduate Nursing Program			$40,982.00 (gained)
Open learning Agency of Australia Meeting Information Needs: Open Learning and Information Literacy	$50,863.25 (gained)		
Committee for the Advancement of University Teaching (DEET) Using Excelcare to Transform Clinical Learning for Undergraduate Nursing Students			$41,769.00 (applied)

20. Certification - to be signed by all applicants

I/We certify that all the details on this form are correct and complete.

I/We understand and agree that:

- research which involves human subjects or experimentation on animals must be carried out in accordance with the guidelines laid down in the NH&MRC Codes of Practice;
- research which involves the use of recombinant nucleic acids constructed in vitro from sources which do not ordinarily recombine genetic information must be carried out in accordance with the guidelines laid down by the Recombinant DNA Monitoring Committee;
- research which involves the use of ionising radiation must have the risks involved assessed by a recognised Ethics, Safety or Bio-safety Committee, and personnel must be trained and hold a current licence, as appropriate; and
- a certificate of compliance with appropriate guidelines must be received from a recognised Ethics, Safety or Bio-safety Committee before payment of any proposed grant can be made.

I/We declare that all persons listed as Associate Investigators have agreed to take part in the proposed research.

Signature of Chief Investigators

1.   Signature

Date   I/We authorise   _____

to sign all subsequent documentation

behalf   Date

/   /

2.   Signature

　　　　　　　　　　　Date

　　　　　　　　　　　　　　　　　　　　　　　　　　/　　　　/

3.   Signature

　　　　　　　　　　　Date

　　　　　　　　　　　　　　　　　　　　　　　　　　/　　　　/

Note: All certificates must be signed.

21.   Certification by Head of School

I certify that the project can be accommodated within the general facilities in my School, and that sufficient working and office space is available for any proposed additional staff. I am prepared to have the project carried out in my School under the circumstances set out by the applicant/s.

I have noted the amount of time which the investigator/s will be devoting to the project and certify that it is appropriate to existing workloads.

Note: A confidential statement may be forwarded to the Grants Sub-Committee

Signature

　　　　　　　　　　　　　　　Date

Name (in block letters):　　　　　　　Designation:

22.   Certification by Director of Centre (CRC, Key, Special) if appropriate for ARC Small Grants only.

I certify that the project cannot be more appropriately accommodated within the Centre's Commonwealth funded research program, but if the application is successful, sufficient working and office space will be made available for the proposed research proposal. I am prepared to have the project carried out as a stand alone project in the Centre under the circumstances set out by the applicant/s.

I have noted the amount of time which the investigator/s will be devoting to the project and certify that it is appropriate to existing workloads.

Signature

Date

Name (in block letters):

Designation:

23.   Aims, research plan, justification of budget, and publications

To answer this question fully, you may wish to refer to the 'Guidelines for 1996 ARC Large Research Grants' so that you can cover the points specifically made in it, especially in relation to policy and priority information and detailed justification of the budget proposal. A copy of these guidelines is available from the Research Office.

Your explanation should be comprehensive but brief.

No more than 13 pages, including this form (but excluding publications), will be considered in the assessment process.

Pages in excess will be discarded.

Use the following headings to detail your answer:

*   Aims and significance
*   Research plan, methods and techniques
*   Progress Report , where project has already commenced
*   Justification of Budget
*   Timetable
*   Benefits of research
*   Plans to apply for external funds to continue the project (Research Development Grant only)
*   Publications - you should list all your refereed publications for the last 5 years. Use asterisks to identify publications relevant to this project.

Where the cooperation or assistance of another body is needed for the project to be successful, the Grants Sub-Committee must be provided with appropriate details.

Appendix B

RESULTS PHASE 1-QUANTITATIVE ANALYSIS OF DATA

Table 1 Type of Print Media

Value Label	Value	Frequency	Valid percent	Cum. percent
Advertiser	1	34	50.0	50.0
Australian Women's Weekly	2	6	8.8	58.8
Dolly	3	16	23.5	82.4
Cleo	4	12	17.6	100.0

Table 2 Year of Publication

Value label	Value	Frequency	Valid percent	Cum. percent
1980	2	3	4.4	4.4
1981	3	12	17.6	22.1
1982	4	4	5.9	27.9
1983	5	5	7.4	35.3
1984	6	1	1.5	36.8
1985	7	6	8.8	45.6
1986	8	2	2.9	48.5
1987	9	1	1.5	50.0
1989	11	8	11.8	61.8
1990	12	1	1.5	63.2
1991	13	1	1.5	64.7
1992	14	1	1.5	66.2
1993	15	1	1.5	67.6
1994	16	5	7.4	75.0
1995	17	17	25.0	100.0

Table 3 Month of Publication

Value Label	Value	Frequency	Valid percent	Cum. percent
January	1	7	10.3	10.3
February	2	5	7.4	17.6
March	3	11	16.2	33.8
April	4	6	8.8	42.6
May	5	7	10.3	52.9
June	6	6	8.8	61.8
July	7	9	13.2	75.0
August	8	5	7.4	82.4
September	9	1	1.5	83.8
October	10	6	8.8	92.6
November	11	3	4.4	97.1
December	12	2	2.9	100.0

Table 4 Day of publication

Value Label	Value	Frequency	Valid percent	Cum. percent
Monday	1	3	8.8	8.8
Tuesday	2	7	20.6	29.4
Wednesday	3	6	17.6	47.1
Thursday	4	2	5.9	52.9
Friday	5	5	14.7	67.6
Saturday	6	11	32.4	100.0
	9	34	Missing	

Table 5 Visual Material

Value Label	Value	Frequency	Valid percent	Cum. percent
Anatomical Drawings	1	3	15.0	15.0
Photos of victims	2	7	35.0	50.0
Photos of families of victims	3	5	25.0	75.0
Sanitary products	4	2	10.0	85.0
General female images	5	2	10.0	95.0
Women exercising	6	1	5.0	100.0
	9	54	Missing	

Table 6 Position in the Paper/Magazine

Value	Value	Frequency	Valid percent	Cum. percent
Headline/leading story	1	2	2.9	2.9
Feature article	2	11	16.2	19.1
Medical advice column	3	15	22.1	42.2
Women's pages	4	2	2.9	44.1
Medical information column	5	4	5.9	50.0
World news	6	7	10.3	60.3
General news item	7	20	29.4	89.7
Contents pages	8	1	1.5	91.2
Special feature by Johnson & Johnson	9	6	8.8	100.0

Table 7 Page number by Media type

	Pages 1-10	Pages 11-40	Pages 41-
Advertiser	25	9	0
Women's Weekly	0	1	5
Dolly	1	0	14
Cleo	2	3	7

Table 8 Position of Article on Page

Value Label	Value	Frequency	Valid percent	Cum. percent
Entire Page	1	9	13.2	13.2
Top left	2	13	19.1	32.4
Top centre	3	3	4.4	36.8
Top right	4	8	11.8	48.5
Left centre	5	3	4.4	52.9
Central	6	7	10.3	63.2
Right central	7	3	4.4	67.6
Bottom left	8	8	11.8	79.4
Bottom central	9	5	7.4	86.8
Bottom right	10	9	13.2	100.0

Table 9 Article Prominence

Value	Value	Frequency	Valid percent	Cum. percent
High	1	40	58.8	58.8
Low	2	28	41.2	100.0

Table 10 Headline Size

Value Label	Value	Frequency	Valid percent	Cum. percent
Small	1	30	44.8	44.8
Medium	2	17	25.4	70.1
Large	3	17	25.4	95.5
Extra large	4	3	4.5	100.0
	9	3	Missing	

Table 11 Style of Print used for Headline

Value Label	Value	Frequency	Valid percent	Cum. percent
Normal	1	50	74.6	74.6
Italics	2	6	9.0	83.6
In negative	3	3	4.5	88.1
Mixed	4	8	11.9	100.0
	9	3	Missing	

Table 12 Headline in Bold

Value	Value	Frequency	Valid percent	Cum. percent
Yes	1	39	58.2	58.2
No	2	28	41.8	100.0
	9	3	Missing	

Table 13 Content of Headlines

Value Label	Value	Frequency	Valid percent	Cum. percent
TSS as a killer disease	1	6	8.0	8.0
TSS as associated with tampon use	2	5	6.7	14.7
TSS as caused by tampon use	3	14	18.7	33.3
TSS as unrelated to tampon use	4	5	6.7	40.0
TSS as a problem of tampon production	5	1	1.3	41.3
TSS as a unknown quantity	6	5	6.7	48.0
TSS as a known quantity	7	4	5.3	53.3
TSS as a disease of tampon hygiene	8	1	1.3	54.7
TSS as a disease that the individual can prevent	9	5	6.7	61.3
Tampons are safe	10	2	2.7	64.0
Tampons are dangerous	11	12	16.0	80.0
TSS and Peta Ann Devine	12	2	2.7	82.7
TSS as a serious condition	13	2	2.7	85.3
TSS as questionable	14	3	4.0	89.3
Neutral	15	4	5.3	94.7
Other	16	4	5.3	100.0
	99	3	Missing	

Table 14 Topic of Article

Value Label	Value	Frequency	Valid Percent	Cum. Percent
TSS as a tampon related disease of unknown origins	1	2	1.6	1.6
General information	2	12	9.8	11.5
Overseas TSS deaths	3	6	4.9	16.4
TSS as caused by Rely tampons	4	6	4.9	21.3
TSS as caused by Carefree tampons	5	3	2.5	23.8
Tampon hygiene	6	14	11.5	35.2
TSS as a staph. infection occurring in both sexes	7	7	5.7	41.0
TSS as a disease of tampon retention	8	11	9.0	50.0
TSS as a disease of tampon production	9	7	5.7	55.7
TSS as a disease of tampon insertion	10	3	2.5	58.2
TSS as a disease arising from super-absorbent tampons	11	5	4.1	62.3
TSS as a bacterial infection	12	10	8.2	70.5
TSS as caused by a lack of anti-bodies to bacterial infection	13	3	2.5	73.0
Peta Ann Devine's inquest	14	7	5.7	78.7
Standards for tampon production	15	7	5.7	84.4
TSS information service	16	2	1.6	86.1
TSS as a bacterial infection transmitted on women's hands	17	1	0.8	86.9
TSS as a waning problem	18	1	0.8	87.7
TSS as unrelated to tampon production	19	3	2.5	90.2
Legal proceedings against tampon producers	20	12	9.8	100.0

Table 15 Content of Lead Sentence

Value Label	Value	Frequency	Valid percent	Cum. percent
TSS as caused by overseas tampons	1	5	5.3	5.3
TSS as a killer disease	2	15	16.0	21.3
TSS as a disease of both sexes	3	5	5.3	26.6
TSS as associated with tampons	4	11	11.7	38.3
TSS as caused by tampons	5	5	5.3	43.6
TSS as not caused by tampons	6	3	3.2	46.8
TSS as a bacterial/golden staph. infection	7	4	4.3	51.1
TSS as a disease of women	8	3	3.2	54.3
TSS as a disease of tampon retention	9	3	3.2	57.4
TSS as a disease of tampon production	10	5	5.3	62.8
TSS as an unknown quantity	11	3	3.2	66.0
TSS as a known quantity	12	2	2.1	68.1
TSS and Australian women	13	3	3.2	71.3
Tampon safety	14	9	9.6	80.9
TSS as a treatable disease	15	2	2.1	83.0
TSS and Peta Ann Devine	16	5	5.3	88.3
TSS as unrelated to tampon production	17	3	3.2	91.5
Other	18	8	8.5	100.00

Table 16 Tone of the Article

Value Label	Value	Frequency	Valid percent	Cum percent
Critical	1	4	3.4	3.4
Regulatory	2	25	21.6	25.0
Expert	3	26	22.4	47.4
Dismissive	4	10	8.6	56.0
Informative	5	35	30.2	86.2
Personalised	6	8	6.9	93.1
Sensational	7	6	5.2	98.3
Speculative	8	1	0.9	99.1
Reassuring	9	1	0.9	100.0

Table 17 Headline Tone

Value Label	Value	Frequency	Valid percent	Cum. percent
Shock	1	15	16.0	16.0
Discreditory	2	5	5.3	21.3
Neutral	3	6	6.4	27.7
Reassuring	4	5	5.3	33.0
Bizarre	5	7	7.4	40.4
Poignant	6	3	3.2	43.6
Informative	7	26	27.7	71.3
Warning	8	17	18.1	89.4
Speculative	9	7	7.4.	96.8
Legal	10	3	3.2	100.0
	99	3	Missing	

Table 18 Sources Quoted in Article

Value Label	Value	Frequency	Valid percent	Cum. percent
Local med/scientist	1	11	12.9	12.9
International med/scientist	2	12	14.1	27.1
NH&MRC	3	7	8.2	35.3
Johnson & Johnson	4	8	9.4	44.7
Victim	5	2	2.4	47.1
Family and friends of victim	6	8	9.4	56.5
Ministerial release	7	5	5.9	62.4
Legal expert	8	6	7.1	69.4
Centre for Disease Control	9	5	5.9	75.3
Standards Association of Australia	10	1	1.2	76.5
Toxic Shock Information Service	11	3	3.5	80.0
Health commission/department	12	4	4.7	84.7
Nurse	13	1	1.2	85.9
Red Cross	14	1	1.2	87.1
Trade practices commission	15	1	1.2	88.2
Therapeutic goods administration	16	1	1.2	89.4
Australian consumer association	17	1	1.2	90.6
Coroner	18	3	3.5	94.1
Food and Drug administration	19	2	2.4	96.5
Women's health centre	20	1	1.2	97.6
Feminist writers	21	1	1.2	98.8
Family planning association	22	1	1.2	100.0
	99	29	Missing	

Table 19 Sources-Social Position

Value Label	Value	Frequency	Valid percent	Cum. percent
Medical system	1	42	49.4	49.4
Industry	2	8	9.4	58.8
Consumer/Victims	3	12	14.1	72.9
Government departments	4	12	14.1	87.1
Legal system	5	9	10.6	97.6
Feminists	6	2	2.4	100.0

Table 20 Relationship to Other Printed Material

Value label	Value	Frequency	Valid percent	Cum. percent
Print once	1	52	74.3	74.3
Reuter	2	5	7.1	81.4
Australian associated press	3	1	1.4	82.9
Medical Journal	4	3	4.3	87.1
Warning from US tampon packet	5	1	1.4	88.6
Research report	6	6	8.6	97.1
Other print media	7	1	1.4	98.6
Feminist books	8	1	1.4	100.0

Table 21 Theoretical or Practical?

Value Label	Value	Frequency	Valid percent	Cum. percent
Theoretical	1	25	36.8	36.8
Practical	2	8	11.8	48.5
Both	3	24	35.3	83.6
Neither	4	11	16.2	100.0

Table 22 Theoretical or Practical Focus by Media Type

	Theoretical	Practical	Both	Neither	**Total**
Advertiser	16	2	5	11	34
Women's Weekly	3	0	3	0	6
Dolly	3	5	8	0	16
Cleo	3	1	8	0	12
Total	25	8	24	11	68

Table 23 Type of Audience pitched at

Value Label	Value	Frequency	Valid percent	Cum. percent
General	1	28	41.2	41.2
Menstruating women	2	6	8.8	50.0
Teenage girls	3	16	23.5	73.5
Women 25 and over	4	6	8.8	82.4
Women 20-40	5	12	17.6	100.0

Table 24 Responsibility for Toxic Shock Syndrome

Value Label	Value	Frequency	Valid percent	Cum. percent
Individual responsibility	1	24	22.6	22.6
Tampon production	2	19	17.9	40.6
Unrelated to tampons	3	10	9.4	50.0
Tampon related of unknown origin	4	11	10.4	60.4
Related to tampons-no blame assigned	5	15	14.2	74.5
Other	6	27	25.5	100.0

Table 25 Responsibility for Toxic Shock by Year

	Individual responsibility	Tampon Production	Unrelated to tampons	Tampon related of unknown origin	Tampon related No blame assigned	Other
1980	0	2	0	0	1	2
1981	5	1	2	6	1	5
1982	1	1	1	1	1	2
1983	1	0	2	0	1	1
1984	0	0	0	0	1	0
1985	4	0	0	2	1	1
1986	1	1	1	1	0	0
1987	1	0	1	0	0	0
1989	1	4	3	0	0	1
1990	0	1	0	0	0	1
1991	1	0	0	0	0	0
1992	1	0	0	0	0	1
1993	1	0	0	0	1	0
1994	3	4	0	0	3	0
1995	2	4	0	0	4	12

Table 26 Subtextual themes by year.

	TSS and Death	TSS and tampons	TSS and bacteria	TSS information	TSS and legal
1980	2	2	0	1	0
1981	1	8	2	4	1
1982	1	1	3	1	1
1983	0	2	3	2	0
1984	0	1	0	0	0
1985	1	5	3	0	0
1986	0	2	1	0	0
1987	0	1	1	0	0
1989	1	8	0	0	5
1990	0	1	0	1	0
1991	0	1	0	0	0
1992	0	1	0	1	0
1993	0	1	1	0	0
1994	0	5	3	1	0
1995	0	6	4	5	7

References

Abercrombie, N., Hill, S. & Turner, B. (Eds.) (1988) *The Penguin Dictionary of Sociology*, 2nd ed., Suffolk, Penguin.

Abraham, A., Knight, C., Mira, M., Frazer, I., McNeil, D. & Llewellyn-Jones, D. (1985) Menstrual Protection: Young Women's Knowledge, Practice and Attitudes, *Journal of Psychosomatic Obstetrics and Gynaecology, 4*, pp.229-236.

Agger, B. (1991) Critical Theory, Post Structuralism, Post Modernism: Their Sociological Relevance, *Annual Review of Sociology, 17*, pp.105-131.

Agger, B. (1992) *Cultural Studies as Critical Theory,* London, Falmer Press.

Albert, E. (1986) Acquired Immune Deficiency Syndrome: The Victim and the Press, *Studies in Communication, 3*, pp.135-158.

Ang, I. & Hermes, J. (1996) Gender and/in Media Consumption, in I. Ang (ed.), *Living Room Wars: Rethinking Media Audiences for a Postmodern World* London, Routledge, pp.109-129.

Armstrong, D. (1985) The Subject and the Social in Medicine: An Appreciation of Michel Foucault, *Sociology of Health and Illness, 7*(1), pp.108-117.

A Schoolgirl's Last Moments (1995, May 24) *The Advertiser,* p.4.

Backhouse, P. (1996) Social Constructionism and its Relevance to Health Policy, *Annual Review of Health Social Sciences, 6*, pp.173-202.

Ball, S. (1990) Introducing Monsieur Foucault, in S. J. Ball (Ed.), *Foucault and Education: Disciplines and Knowledge*, London, Routledge, pp.1-8.

Bakhtin, M. (1981) *The Dialogic Imagination: Four Essays by Mikhail Bakhtin,* Austin, University of Texas Press.

Bail, K., Murray-Smith, A. & Shaw, J. (1985) Dolly: A Girl Like Who? A Reading of *Dolly* Magazine, *Melbourne Journal of Politics, 17,* pp.85-109.

Baird, B. & Sheridan, S. (1992) Indexing the Australian Women's Weekly, *The Australian Library Journal,* May, pp.145-150.

Bartky, S. (1988) Foucault, Femininity, and the Modernization of Patriarchal Power, in I. Diamond & L. Quinby (Eds.), *Feminism and Foucault: Reflections on Resistance*, Boston, Northeastern University Press, pp.61-68.

Bauman, Z. (1992) *Intimations of Postmodernity*, London, Routledge.

Beattie, J., Cheek, J. & Gibson, T. (1996) The Politics of Collaboration as Viewed Through the Lens of a Collaborative Research Project, *Journal of Advanced Nursing, 24*, pp.682-687.

Bell, P., Boehringer, K. & Crofts, S. (1982) *Programmed Politics: A Study of Australian Television*, Sydney, Sable.

Bertens, H. (1995) *The Idea of the Postmodern: A History*, London, Routledge.

Best, S. & Kellner, D. (1991) *Postmodern Theory: Critical Interrogations*, New York, Guilford Press.

Block Coutts, L. & Berg, D. (1993) The Portrayal of the Menstruating Women in Menstrual Products Advertisements, *Health Care for Women International, 14*, pp.179-191.

Bloland, H. (1995) Postmodernism and Higher Education, *Journal of Higher Education, 66*(5), pp.521-559.

Brewer, J.D. (1994) The Ethnographic Critique of Ethnography: Sectarianism in the RUC, *Sociology, 28*(1), pp.231-244.

Brink, P. & Wood, M. (1994) *Basic Steps in Planning Nursing Research: From Question to Proposal* (4th ed.) Boston, Jones & Bartlett publishers.

Brooks, A. (1994, August) How to Beat Period Panic, *Dolly*, pp.104-5.

Brooks, A. (1995, July) Toxic Shock Report, *Dolly*, pp.54-56.

Brown, C. & Seddon, J. (1996) Nurses, Doctors and the Body of the Patients: Medical Dominance Revisited, *Nursing Inquiry, 3*(1), pp.30-35.

Burrell, G. (1988) Modernism, Post Modernism and Organizational Analysis 2: The Contribution of Michel Foucault, *Organizational Studies, 9*, pp.221-235.

Burman, E. (1992) Developmental Psychology and the Postmodern Child, in J. Doherty, E. Graham and M. Malek (eds) *Postmodernism and the Social Sciences*, New York, Macmillan.

Cheek, J. (1995a) Nurses, Nursing and Representation: An Exploration of the Effect of Viewing Positions on the Textual Portrayal of Nursing, *Nursing Inquiry, 2*, pp.235-240.

Cheek, J. (1995b) (Re)viewing Health: Textual Representations of Aspects of Contemporary Australian Health Care, *Australian Journal of Communication, 22*(3), pp.52-62.

Cheek, J. (1996) Taking a View: Qualitative Research as Representation, *Qualitative Health Research, 6*(4), pp.459-507.

Cheek, J. (1997a) (Con)textualizing Toxic Shock Syndrome: Selected Media Representations of an Emergent Health Phenomenon 1979-1995, *Health, 1*(2), pp.183-203.

Cheek, J. (1997b) Negotiating Delicately: Conversations about Health, *Health and Social Care in the Community, 5*(1), pp.23-7.

Cheek, J. (1997c) Nurses and the Administration of Medication: Broadening the Focus, *Clinical Nursing Research, 6*(3), pp.253-274

Cheek, J. (1997d) Postmodern Theory and Nursing: Simply Talking Trivialities in High-sounding Language, in H. Keleher & F. McInerney (eds.), *Nursing Matters* Churchill Livingstone, Melbourne, pp.79-95.

Cheek, J & Gibson, T. (1996) The Discursive Construction of the Role of the Nurse in Medication Administration: An Exploration of the Literature, *Nursing Inquiry, 3*, pp.83-90.

Cheek, J., & Gibson, T. (1997) Policy Matters: Critical Policy Analysis and Nursing, *Journal of Advanced Nursing*, 25, pp.668-672.

Cheek, J. & Porter, S. (1997) Reviewing Foucault: Possibilities and Problems for Nursing and Health Care, *Nursing Inquiry, 4*, pp.108-119.

Cheek, J., & Rudge, T. (1993) The Power of Normalisation: Foucauldian Perspectives on Contemporary Health Care Practices, *Australian Journal of Social Issues, 28*(4), pp.271-284.

Cheek, J. & Rudge, T. (1994a) *Advanced Practice Studies 3, Nursing Practice as Textually Mediated Reality,* Underdale, University of South Australia.

Cheek, J. & Rudge, T. (1994b) Inquiry into Nursing as Textually Mediated Discourse, in P. Chinn (ed.), *Advances in Methods of Inquiry for Nursing* Gaithsburg, Aspen Publishers, pp.59-67.

Cheek, J. & Rudge, T. (1994c) Nursing as Textually Mediated Reality, *Nursing Inquiry, 1*(1), pp.15-22.

Cheek, J., & Rudge, T. (1994d) The Panopticon Revisited?: An Exploration of the Social and Political Dimensions of Contemporary Health Care and Nursing Practice, *International Journal of Nursing Studies, 31*(6), pp.583-591.

Cheek, J. & Rudge, T. (1994e) Webs of Documentation: The Discourse of Case Notes, *Australian Journal of Communication, 21*(2), pp.41-52.

Cheek, J., Shoebridge, J., Willis, E & Zadoroznyj, M. (1996) *Society and Health: Social Theory for Health Workers.* Melbourne, Longman Cheshire.

Chia, R. (1996) The Problem of Reflexivity in Organizational Research: Towards a Postmodern Science of Organization, *Organization, 3*(1), 31-59.

Chrisler, J. & Levy, K. (1990) The Media Constructs a Menstrual Monster: A Content Analysis of PMS Articles in Popular Press, *Women and Health, 16*(2), pp.89-104.

Cixous, H. (1986) Sorties, in H Cixous & C. Clement (eds.), *The Newly Born Woman* Manchester, Manchester University Press, pp.63-129.

Clarke, J. N. (1991) Media Portrayal of Disease from the Medical, Political, Economy, and Lifestyle Perspectives, *Qualitative Health Research, 1*(3), pp.287-308.

Colbry, S. L. (1992) A Review of Toxic Shock Syndrome: The Need for Education Still Exists, *Nurse Practitioner, 17*(9), pp.39-46.

Collins, R. (1990) Cumulation and Anti-cumulation in Sociology, *American Sociological Review, 55*, pp.462-463.

Collyer, F. (1996) Understanding Ulcers: Medical Knowledge, Social Constructionism, and Helicobacter Pylori, *Annual Review of Health Social Sciences, 6*, pp.1-40.

Could You Please Explain What Toxic Shock Syndrome Is? (1985, May) *Dolly,* p.137.

Craik, J. (1989) Cleo's Age of Consent, *Australian Left Review,* 111, pp.37-38.

Dalley, G. (1988) *Ideologies of Caring: Rethinking Community and Collectivism,* Basingstoke, Macmillan Educational.

Daniel, S. (1995) Postmodernity, Poststructuralism, and the Historiography of Modern Philosophy, *International Philosophical Quarterly, Vol. XXXV*, 3, Issue 139, pp.255-267.

Davies, B. (1989) *Frogs and Snails and Feminist Tales,* Sydney, Allen and Unwin.

Dean, M. (1994) *Critical and Effective Histories: Foucault's Methods and Historical Sociology,* London, Routledge.

Delaney, J., Lupton, M. J. & Toth, E. (1988) *The Curse: A Cultural History of Menstruation,* Champaign, IL, University of Illinois Press.

De Montigney, G. A. J. (1995) The Power of Being Professional, in M. Campbell & A. Manicom (eds.), *Knowledge, Experience and Ruling Relations: Studies in the Social Organization of Knowledge* Toronto, University of Toronto, pp.209-220.

Denzin, N. (1989) *The Research Act,* Chicago, Aldine.

Denzin, N. (1994) Postmodernism and Deconstruction, in D. Dickens & A. Fontana (eds), *Postmodernism and Social Inquiry* New York, Guilford, pp.182-202.

Denzin, N., & Lincoln, Y. (1994) Entering the Field of Qualitative Research, in N. Denzin & Y. Lincoln (eds.), *Handbook of Qualitative Research* California, Sage, pp.1-18.

Derrida, J. (1976) *Of Grammatology*, Gayatri Chakrovorty Spivak (Trans.) Baltimore, John Hopkins University Press.

Dzurec, L. (1989) The Necessity for and Evolution of Multiple Paradigms for Nursing Research: A Poststructuralist Perspective. *Advances in Nursing Science, 11*(4), pp.69-77.

Eagleton, T. (1983) *Literary Theory: An introduction*, Minneapolis, University of Minnesota Press.

Fairclough, N. (1992) Discourse and Text: Linguistic and Intertextual Analysis within Discourse Analysis, *Discourse and Society, 3*(2), pp.193-217.

Feldman, M (1995*) Strategies for Interpreting Qualitative Data,* Thousand Oaks, Sage.

Fischer, H. & Skondras, H. (1993) Social Responsibility: The Case of Women's Sanitary Products, *Wisenet, 33*, pp.14-17.

Foster, H. (1985) Postmodernism: A Preface, in *Postmodern Culture*, (pp.ix-xvi) London, Pluto Press.

Foucault, M. (1974) *The Archaeology of Knowledge,* London, Tavistock.

Foucault, M (1975) *The Birth of the Clinic*, New York, Vintage Books.

Foucault, M. (1977) *Discipline and Punish*, London, Tavistock.

Foucault, M (1979) Governmentality, *I & C, 5*, pp.5-21.

Foucault, M. (1980) *Power/Knowledge*, C. Gordon (Ed.) Brighton, Harvester Press.

Foucault, M. (1982) Afterword: The Subject and Power, in H Dreyfus and P. Rabinow (eds.), *Michel Foucault: Beyond Structuralism and Hermeneutics*, Chicago, University of Chicago Press, pp.208-226.

Foucault, M. (1984) The Order of Discourse, in M. Shapiro (ed.), *Language and Politics* Oxford, Basil Blackwell, pp.108-38.

Fowler, R. (1991) *Language in the News: Discourse and Ideology*, London, Routledge.

Fox, N. (1991) Postmodernism, Rationality and the Evaluation of Health Care, *Sociological Review, 39*(2), pp.709-744.

Fox, N. (1993a) Discourse, Organisation and the Surgical Ward Round, *Sociology of Health and Illness, 15*(4), pp.16-42.

Fox, N. (1993b) *Postmodernism, Sociology and Health,* Toronto, University of Toronto Press.

Fox, N. (1994) Anaesthetists, the Discourse on Patient Fitness and the Organisation of Surgery, *Sociology of Health and Illness, 16*(1), pp.1-18.

Fox, N. (1995) Postmodern Perspectives on Care: The Vigil and the Gift, *Critical Sociology Today, 15*(2/3), pp.107-125.

Fox, N. (1997) Texts, Frames and Decisions over Discharge from Hospital: A Deconstruction, *Social Sciences in Health: The International Journal of Research and Practice, 3*(1), pp.41-51.

Frazer, E. (1992) Teenage Girls Reading "Jackie", *Media, Culture, Society, 9*, pp.407-425.

Freidson, E. (1970) *Professional Dominance: The Social Structure of Medical Care*, New York, Atherton Press.

Gabe, J., Gustaffason, U. & Bury, M. (1991) Mediating Illness: Newspaper Coverage of Tranquilliser Dependence, *Sociology of Health and Illness, 13*, pp.332-353.

Gameson, J. (1990) Rubber Wars: Struggles over the Condom in the United States, *Journal of the History of Sexuality, 1*(2), pp.262-282.

Garland, S. M. & Peel, M. M. (1995) Tampons and Toxic Shock Syndrome, *The Medical Journal of Australia, 163*, pp.8-9.

Garrett, L. (1994) *The Coming Plague: Newly Emerging Diseases in a World Out of Balance*, New York, Farrar, Straus and Giroux.

Gilbert, T. (1995) Nursing: Empowerment and the Problem of Power, *Journal of Advanced Nursing, 21*, pp.865-871.

Ginsburg, R. (1996) 'Don't Tell, Dear': The Material Culture of Tampons and Napkins, *Journal of Material Culture, 1*(3), pp.365-375.

Giroux, H. (1992) *Border Crossings*, New York, Routledge.

Glaser, B. (1978) *Theoretical Sensitivity – Advances in the Methodology of Grounded Theory*, Mill Valley, Sociology Press.

Glaser, B. (1992) *Basics of Grounded Theory Analysis: Emergence vs Forcing*, Mill Valley, Sociology Press.

Glaser, B. & Strauss, A (1967) *The Discovery of Grounded Theory: Strategies for Qualitative Research*, New York, Aldine.

Gledhill, C. (1988) Pleasurable Negotiations, in E. Pribham (ed.), *Female Spectators: Looking at Film and Television* London, Verso, pp.64-89.

Gouldner, A. (1971) *The Coming Crisis of Western Sociology*, London, Heinemann.

Guillemin, M. (1996) Constructing Menopause: Knowledge Through Socio-material Practices, *Annual Review of Health Social Sciences, 6*, pp.41-56.

Hacking, I. (1991) The Archaeology of Foucault, in D. Hoy (ed.), *Foucault: A Critical Reader* Oxford, Basil Blackwell, pp.27-40.

Hailstone, B. (1981, February 28) Carefree Tampons Cleared of Blame, *The Advertiser*, p.9.

Hall, S. (1982) The Rediscovery of "Ideology". Return of the Repressed in Media Studies, in M. Gurevitch, T. Bennett and J Wollacott (eds.), *Culture, Society and the Media* London, Methuen, pp.30-55.

Hamilton, H. & Gray, G. (1992) *A Guide to Successful Grant Applications: Grant Application Know How*, Melbourne, Royal College of Nursing.

Hampson, N. (1993) Enlightenment, in W. Outhwaite & T. Bottomore (Eds.), *The Blackwell Dictionary of Twentieth Century Social Thought,* Oxford, Blackwell.

Hanrahan, S. N. (1994) Historical Review of Menstrual Toxic Shock Syndrome, *Women & Health, 21* (2/3), pp.141-165.

Hebdige, D. (1988) Hiding in the Light: On Images and Things, London, Comedia.

Hertz, R. (1996) Introduction: Ethics, Reflexivity and Voice, *Qualitative Sociology, 19*(1), pp.3-9.

Hollway, W. (1989) *Subjectivity and Method in Psychology: Gender, Meaning and Science*, London, Sage.

Horsfall, J. (1995) Madness in our Methods: Nursing Research and Epistemology, *Nursing Inquiry, 2*, pp.2-9.

Hoskin, K. (1990) Foucault Under Examination: The Crypto-educationalist Unmasked, in S Ball (ed.), *Foucault and Education: Disciplines and Knowledge,* London, Routledge, pp.29-53.

Hoy, D. (1991a) Introduction, in D. Hoy (ed.), *Foucault: A Critical Reader* Oxford, Basil Blackwell, pp.1-26.

Hoy, D. (1991b) Power, Repression, Progress: Foucault, Lukes and the Frankfurt School, in D Hoy (ed.), *Foucault: A Critical Reader* Oxford, Basil Blackwell, pp.123-148.

I Was Wondering If You Could Give Me Some Information on Toxic Shock Syndrome. (1986, March) *Cleo*, p.11.

Johnson, J. L. (1994) A Dialectical Examination of Nursing Art, *Advances in Nursing Science, 17,* pp.1-14.

Jacobson, S. & Jacques, R. (1997) Destabilizing the Field: Poststructuralist Knowledge-Making Strategies in a Postindustrial Era, *Journal of Management Inquiry, 6*(1), pp.42-59.

Kaplan, M. (1992) *Motherhood and Representation: The Mother in Popular Culture and Melodrama*, New York, Routledge.

Kennedy, A. (1980, October 10th) Tampons - and Toxic Shock, *The Advertiser*, p.29.

Kermode, S. & Brown, C. (1996) The Postmodern Hoax and its Effects on Nursing, *International Journal of Nursing Studies, 33*(4), pp.375-384.

Kerr, S. (1995a, March 18) Death in a Packet, *The Advertiser,* pp.33-34.

Kerr, S. (1995b, March 18) New Move to Ease Tampon Illness Fear, *The Advertiser,* p.26.

Kress, G. (1985) *Linguistic Processes in Socio-cultural Practice*, Victoria, Deakin University Press.

King, H. (1983, March) Toxic Shock in Transsexual, *Cleo*, p.141.

Latimer, J. (1995) The Nursing Process Re-examined: Enrolment and Translation, *The Journal of Advanced Nursing, 22,* pp.213-220.

Lange, A. & Cheek, J. (1997) Health Policy and the Nursing Profession - a Deafening Silence, *International Journal of Nursing Practice, 3,* pp.2-9.

Laws, S. (1990) *Issues of Blood: The Politics of Menstruation*, Houndsmill, Macmillan.

Long, J. (1992) Foucault's Clinic, *Journal of Medical Humanities, 13*(3), pp.119-138.

Lupton, D. (1992) Discourse Analysis: A New Methodology for Understanding the Ideologies of Health and Illness, *Australian Journal of Public Health, 16*(2), pp.145-150.

Lupton, D. (1993) Is There Life after Foucault? Poststructuralism and the Health Social Sciences, *Australian Journal of Public Health, 17*(4), pp.298-300.

Lupton, D. (1994a) Analysing News Coverage, in Chapman, S & Lupton, D. (Eds.), *The Fight for Public Health: Principles and Practice of Media Advocacy*, London, BMJ, pp.23-57.

Lupton, D. (1994b) The Condom in the Age of AIDS: Newly Respectable or Still a Dirty Word? A Discourse Analysis, *Qualitative Health Research, 4*(3), pp.304-320.

Lupton, D. (1994c) Femininity, Responsibility, and the Technological Imperative: Discourses on Breast Cancer in the Australian Press, *International Journal of Health Services, 24*(1), pp.73-89.

Lupton, D. (1994d) *Medicine as Culture: Illness, Disease and the Body in Western Societies*, London, Sage.

Lupton, D. (1995) Anatomy of an 'Epidemic': Press Reporting of an Outbreak of Legionnaire's Disease, *Media Information Australia, 76*, May, pp.92-99.

Lyotard, J. (1984) *The Postmodern Condition: A Report on Knowledge*, Minneapolis, University of Minnesota Press.

MacKenzie, F. (1991, July) Tampon Safety, *The Australian Women's Weekly*, p.117.

May, C. R. & Purkis, M. E. (1995) The Configuration of Nurse-patient Relationships: A Critical View, *Scholarly Inquiry for Nursing Practice*, pp.283-295.

May, C. (1992) Individual Care? Power and Subjectivity in Therapeutic Relationships, *Sociology, 26*, pp.589-602.

May, C., Dowrick, C. & Richardson, M. (1996) The Confidential Patient: The Social Construction of Therapeutic Relationships in General Medical Practice, *Sociological Review, 44*(2), pp.187-203.

McNicoll, D. (1982) The Weekly: A 50-year Phenomenon, *The Bulletin, Oct 12,* pp.40-48.

Miller, P. & Rose, N. (1990) Governing Economic Life, *Economy and Society, 19* (1), pp.1-31.

Mitchell, D. (1996) Postmodernism, Health and Illness, *Journal of Advanced Nursing,* 23, pp.201-5.

Morley, D. (1992) Television, Audiences and Cultural Studies, London, Routledge.

Mullhall, A. (1995) Nursing Research: What Difference Does it Make? *Journal of Advanced Nursing, 21*(3), pp.576-583.

Munday, R. (1981, February 25th) Tampons and Toxic Shock: What You Should Know, *The Australian Women's Weekly,* p.13.

Nelkin, D. (1991) AIDS and the News Media, *The Milbank Quarterly, 69*(2), 293-307.

Nettleton, S. (1991) Wisdom, Diligence and Teeth: Discursive Practices and the Creation of Mothers, *Sociology of Health and Illness, 13*(1), pp.98-111.

Nisbet, R. (1971) *The Degradation the Academic Dogma: The University in America 1945-1970,* Heinemann, London.

Norris, C. (1991) *Deconstruction, Theory and Practice* (Rev. ed.), Routledge, London.

Olesen, V. L. (1986) Analyzing Emergent Issues in Women's Health: The Case of Toxic-Shock Syndrome, in V. L. Olesen & N. F. Woods (Eds.), *Culture, Society, and Menstruation,* New York, Hemisphere Publishing Corporation, pp.51-62.

Parker, I. (1992) *Discourse Dynamics: Critical Analysis for Social and Individual Psychology,* London, Routledge.

Parker, J. & Wiltshire, J. (1995) The Handover: Three Modes of Nursing Practice Knowledge, in G Gray & R Pratt (eds.) *Scholarship in the Discipline of Nursing* Melbourne, Churchill Livingstone, pp.151-168.

Parton, N. (1994) The Nature of Social Work Under the Conditions of Postmodernity, *Social Work and Social Sciences Review, 5*(2), pp.93-112.

Philp, M. (1985) Michel Foucault, in Q Skinner (ed.), *The Return of Grand Theory in the Human Sciences* Cambridge, Cambridge University Press, pp.65-81.

Poirer, S. & Brauner, D. (1990) The Voices of the Medical Record, *Theoretical Medicine, 11,* pp.29-39.

Popper, K. (1976) Reason or Revolution, in R. Adorno, R. Dahrendorf, J. Habermas, H. Pilot & K. Popper (eds.), *The Positivist Dispute in German Sociology,* Heinemann, London, pp.288-300.

Porter, S. (1993) Nursing Research Conventions: Objectivity or Obfuscation? *Journal of Advanced Nursing, 18,* pp.137-143.

Porter, S. (1997) The Degradation of the Academic Dogma, *Journal of Advanced Nursing, 25,* pp.655-656.

Price, K. (1996) Nursing, Pain and Pain Management, *Nursing Inquiry, 4,* pp.72-73.

Price, K & Cheek, J. (1996a) Exploring the Nursing Role in Pain Management from a Post-structuralist Perspective, *Joumal of Advanced Nursing, 24,* pp.899-904.

Price, K. & Cheek, J. (1996b) Pain as a Discursive Construction, *Social Sciences in Health, 2*(4), pp.211 - 217.

Purkis, M. E. (1994) Representations of Action: Reorienting Field Studies in Nursing Practice, in P.Chinn (ed.) *Advances in Methods of Inquiry for Nursing* Gaithsburg, Aspen, pp.13-31.

Rabinow, P. (1984) Introduction, in P. Rabinow (ed.) *The Foucault Reader* Pantheon, New York, pp.3-29.

Reid, K. (1991) Thompson V. Johnson and Johnson PTY LTD, *Melbourne University Law Review, 18*, (June), pp.182-185.

Rice, P. (1989, August 8) Tampons 'Not Linked' to Toxic Shock, *The Advertiser*, p.8.

Richardson, L. (1994) Writing: A Method of Inquiry, in N. Denzin and Y Lincoln (Eds), *Handbook of Qualitative Research* Sage, California, pp.516-529.

Ripper, M. (1991) *The Engendering of Hormones: The Role of the Menstrual Cycle and its Disorders in the Contemporary Construction of Gender*, unpublished doctoral dissertation, Flinders University, Adelaide.

Romanyshyn, R. (1989) *Technology as a Symptom and Dream*, London, Routledge.

Rosenau, P. (1992) *Post-modernism and the Social Sciences: Insights, Inroads and Intrusions*, Princeton, New Jersey, Princeton University Press.

Rosenau, P. (1994) Revitalizing Sociology: Post Modern Perspectives on Methodology, *Current Perspectives in Social Theory, 14*, pp.89-99.

Russell, C. (1993) Hype, Hysteria, and Women's Health Risks: The Role of the Media, *Women's Health Issues, 3*(4), pp.191-197.

Sacks, V. (1996) Women and AIDS: An Analysis of Media Misrepresentations, *Social Science and Medicine, 42*(1), pp.59-73.

Sanders, N. (1988) Angels on the Image, in G Kress (ed.), *Communication and Culture: An Introduction* Kensington, University of New South Wales Press, pp.131-156.

Sarup, M. (1989) *An Introductory Guide to Post-structuralism and Postmodernism*, Athens, The University of Georgia Press.

Schutt, R. (1996) *Investigating the Social World: The Process and Practice of Research*, Thousand Oaks, California, Pine Forge Press.

Short, S. (1996) Editorial, *Annual Review of Health Social Sciences*, 6, p.v.

Silverman, D. & Gubruim, J. (1989) Introduction, in J. Gubrium J. & D. Silverman, (Eds.), *The Politics of Field Research: Sociology Beyond Enlightenment* London, Sage, pp.1-12.

Smart, B. (1991) The Politics of Truth and the Problem of Hegemony, in D. Hoy (ed.), *Foucault: A Critical Reader* Oxford, Basil Blackwell, pp.157-174.

Smart, B. (1992) *Modern Conditions, Postmodern Controversies*, Routledge, London.

Spivak, G. C. (1976) Translators preface, in Gayatri Chakrovorty Spivak (Trans.) *Of Grammatology*, Baltimore, John Hopkins University Press.

Squier, S. (1993) Representing the Reproductive Body, *Meridian* 12(1), pp.29-45.

Stallings, R. (1990) Media Discourse and the Social Construction of Risk, *Social Problems, 37*(1), pp.80-95.

Stone, J. (1991) Contextualizing Biogenetic and Reproductive Technologies, *Critical Studies in Mass Communication*, 8, pp.309-332.

Street, A. (1997) Thinking about Nursing Futures, *Nursing Inquiry*, 4(2), p.79.

Strauss, A. & Corbin, J. (1990) *Basics of Qualitative Research Grounded Theory Procedures and Techniques*, Newbury Park, Sage.

Tampons (1985, October) *Dolly*, p.154.

Tampon Warning (1980, October 7) *The Advertiser*, p.2.

The Macquarie Dictionary (1985) West End, Queensland, Herron publications.

Thomas, C. (1993) Deconstructing Concepts of Care, *Sociology, 27*, pp.649-70.

Thompson, C. & Hirschman, E. (1995) Understanding the Socialized Body: A Poststructuralist Analysis of Consumer's Self-conceptions, Body Images, and Self-care Practices, *Journal of Consumer Research, 22*, pp.139-153.

Thompson, K. (1992) Social Pluralism and Post-modernity, in S. Hall, D. Held & T. McGrew (eds), *Modernity and its Futures* Cambridge, Polity Press, pp.222-256.

Toxic Shock Victim No.4 Discharged (1981, March 31st) *The Advertiser,* p.6.

T.S.S: Mystery Disease Linked with Tampons (1981, February) *Cleo,* pp.118-9.

Turner, B. (1987) *Medical Power and Social Knowledge,* London, Tavistock.

Turner, R. (1989) Deconstructing the Field, in J. Gubrium J. & D. Silverman, (Eds.), *The Politics of Field Research: Sociology Beyond Enlightenment* London, Sage, pp.13-19.

Van Dijk, T. (1997) Editorial: Analysing Discourse Analysis, *Discourse and Society,* 8(1), pp.5-6.

Wajcman, J. (1994) Technological A/Genders: Technology, Culture and Class, in L. Green & R. Guinery (eds.), *Framing Technology: Society, Choice and Change,* St. Leonards, NSW, Allen & Unwin, pp.3-14.

Waltzer, M. (1988) *The Company of Critics,* New York: Basic Books.

Watson, J. (1995) Postmodernism and Knowledge Development in Nursing, *Nursing Science Quarterly, 8*(2), pp.60-64.

Weaver, A. (1994) Deconstructing Dirt and Disease: The Case of TB, in M. Bloor & P. Taraborrelli (eds.), *Qualitative Studies in Health and Medicine* Avebury, Ashgate Publishing, pp.76-95.

Weedon, C. (1987) *Feminist Practice and Post Structuralist Theory,* London, Basil Blackwell.

Whitworth, J. (1994) The Direction of Medical Research in Australia, *Collegian, 1*(1), pp.26-28.

Wicks, D. (1995) Nurses and Doctors and Discourses of Healing, *Australian and New Zealand Journal of Sociology, 31*(2), pp.122-139.

Wilson , P. (1980, June 2) "Scary" New Disease Kills Women, *The Advertiser,* p.1.

Winston, B. (1990) On Counting the Wrong Things, in M. Alvardo & J. B. Thompson (Eds.), *The Media Reader,* London, British Film Institute, pp.50-64.

Woman in Vic. Has Tampon Infection (1981, January, 30th) *The Advertiser*, p.1.

Woman Sues Tampon Maker (1989, July 25th) *The Advertiser*, p.5.

Workman, T. (1996) *Banking on Deception: The Discourse of Fiscal Crisis,* Halifax, Fernwood Publishing.

Wright, J. (1982, April 7th) Preventing Toxic Shock. *The Australian Women's Weekly,* p.93.

Yoxen, E. (1985) Licensing Reproductive Technologies? *Issues in Radical Science, 17,* pp.138-148.

Index

About the Author

Professor Julianne Cheek is internationally recognised for her expertise in qualitative research in health related areas. She is currently Dean of the Research Division of Health Sciences, University of South Australia and Director of the Centre for Research into Nursing and Health Care, which is a university designated and funded performance-based research centre. She has experienced outstanding success in attracting funding for qualitative research projects, with some sixteen projects funded in the past four years. She has also attracted large sums of funding for projects related to teaching that have qualitative principles embedded within them.

Professor Cheek has published over 40 refereed book chapters and journal articles, many of which explore the application of postmodern and poststructural approaches to health care. One of the books she coauthored (*Society and Health*) won the prize for the Tertiary Single Book (wholly Australian) in the 1996 Australian Awards for Excellence in Educational Publishing. She has presented more than 40 papers at international and national conferences, including keynote addresses in Vancouver, Canada; Kuala Lumpur, Malaysia; and Queensland, Australia.